We Are Timeless

The Radiance Technique®
in
Hospice Care

Christine Maria Gross

FIRST PORTAL WISDOM PAPERBACK EDITION PUBLISHED 2012

Library and Archives Canada Cataloguing in Publication

Gross, Christine Maria, 1965-
    We are timeless: The Radiance Technique® in hospice care/Christine Maria Gross.

Includes bibliographical references.
ISBN 978-0-9784625-0-5 (pbk.)

    1. Reiki (Healing system). 2. Touch—Therapeutic use. 3. Vibration—Therapeutic use. 4. Hospice care. I. Title.

RZ600.G76 2012   615.8'51   C2008-906426-7
                        CIP

Cover Design by Meredith Karns
Cover Photograph © Courtney Milne, Earth from Space.
Author Photograph © Edward Ambrosius

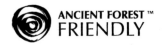

Dedication

to
my mother
for her
compassion, care and love

to
my father
for his
generosity, insight and love

to
Ilse
for her
inspiration, strength and love

and to
Dr. Barbara Ray
for her
wisdom, guidance and love

Praise for *We Are Timeless*

"I have been deeply touched by the beautiful sharings within this book. They come straight from the hearts of those who have had the direct experience of the use of The Radiance Technique® within their own lives."

> ~ DR. BARBARA RAY
> author of *The 'Reiki' Factor in The Radiance Technique*®

"Healing is not an accident. It takes work by the patient and their caregivers and The Radiance Technique® shows us how to make it happen."

> ~ BERNIE S. SIEGEL, M.D.
> author of *Love, Medicine & Miracles* and *Help Me To Heal*

"In this illuminating book, Christine Gross makes us pause and slow down to hear the stories, the words from people all over the world whose lives have been transformed from a unique system and approach that has its roots in ancient practices. If life can be made better, if relief can come from debilitating illness and pain can be achieved and if peace of mind can be given so easily and so seamlessly, then why not reach out for it? Christine shows us the way in a book that takes us on this quiet and meaningful journey."

> ~ MARTY GERVAIS
> Author, Founder Black Moss Press

"This is an extremely important book, not only for hospice workers, but for any healthcare providers interested in alleviating suffering. It is a wonderful introduction to a new realm in the care of patients."

> ~ PAUL DUGLISS, M.D
> author of *Ayurveda – The Power to Heal* and *Yoga and Ayurveda*

"The Radiance Technique® is of great benefit to any person, especially to those patients who are in need of palliative care. This technique is helpful in alleviating their symptoms and supporting a better quality of life."

> ~ DR. HAKAM ABU-ZAHRA
> Medical Oncologist, Windsor Regional Cancer Centre, Canada

"It is very inspiring, encouraging and expanding to read and be with this profound book. Gratitude to the author, Christine Gross, and all who shared selflessly their deep experiences with the Radiant Touch® in a variety of situations in hospice care."

> ~ ULRIKE WOLF
> author of *Die Radiance Technik, Das authentische Reiki,* Germany

"With a sensitivity born of her own journey through cancer to wellness, Christine Maria Gross has written an account of The Radiance Technique® and its uses that are substantiated by clinical research and experience, immediately applicable in medical practices, urgently needed by patients and spiritually profound. Simple, safe and highly effective, The Radiance Technique® should be an integral part of every clinic, hospital and hospice. Indeed, after reading the descriptions of the life-transforming power of this compassionate and humane healing modality, I hope that everyone in every field of medicine has the good fortune to learn, experience and share it with their patients and their families. This book is an important contribution to the field of integrative medicine and holistic healthcare."

~ DAVID CROW, L.AC.
author of *In Search of the Medicine Buddha*

"This is a book that has touched my heart. It is filled with enlightening, compassionate, and timeless stories about Radiant Touch®, a healing form of care giving for people at their end of life. I am so grateful to Christine for bringing awareness to the importance of this technique in support of patients' traditional medical care, their comfort, and quality of life. This book is a gift. I will recommend it to healthcare providers, caretakers, patients, and lay people in hopes that these powerful stories and this comforting technique can make healthcare a kinder and gentler place."

~ ANN WEBSTER, PH.D.
Director Mind Body Program for Cancer
Benson-Henry Institute for Mind Body Medicine, Massachusetts, USA

"This book is a gift to treasure because it gives both hope to those who are living with an illness and a positive non-invasive way to have control of their life's journey. Through this collection of personal experiences, readers will be touched by the comfort and peace Radiant Touch® offers during some of life's most challenging times. Learning this self-help method has been nurturing in my healing and even now, eighteen years later, I continue to use The Radiance Technique®!"

~ SUSAN HESS
Cancer Survivor, Past President Willow Breast Cancer Support Canada

"Christine Gross is an inspiring and compassionate healer and her recommendation for the use of sound within the hospice movement is an essential way forward at this time."

~ JILL PURCE
author of *The Mystic Spiral*
Pioneer of Healing Sound Movement: The Healing Voice

Love is the only Purpose of Life.
Love is the only Reason for Living.
Love is the only Power.
LOVE is All there Is.

~ *Dr. Barbara Ray, Ph.D. with Shoshana Shay, comp.*
'This Moment in Time,' The Awakening Journey® Day by Day,
Selections from the Teachings of Dr. Barbara Ray.

CONTENTS

PART FOUR

PART FIVE

Reader's Note

For the purposes of this book, you will notice that the phrases The Radiance Technique®, Authentic Reiki®, Radiant Touch® or TRT® are used with the correct "®", delineating them as registered service marks. These registered service marks denote this authentic technique and no other. Their use in books such as this is to refer to the actual technique itself. The Radiant TRT Heart First Ashram®, Real Reiki® and The Official Reiki Program® are also registered service marks. All these marks are registered by The Radiance Technique International Association, Inc. (TRTIA) and are held and maintained by that nonprofit organization. Authorized Instructors are given permission to use them specifically, and manuscripts are reviewed for accuracy of usage.

*I am the infinite Ocean
become many in the waves.
I am eternal and immortal.
I am Spirit.*

~ Yogananda

Foreword

It is with great Joy that we have been looking forward to the publication of this book about The Radiance Technique® and the use of Radiant Touch® among hospice clients and those who assist and care for them. This book has certainly been compiled with love and compassion by author Christine Maria Gross and all those who share within these pages how their lives have been expanded by using Radiant Touch®. Their sharings show their pain and their joy, as well as the inspiration they have found through their own deep insights into the process they have been through while using TRT®.

As an Authorized Instructor of The Radiance Technique®, Authentic Reiki®, Christine has chosen to use her profession to reach out with and to serve others, combined with her special skills and training with The Hospice of Windsor and Essex County Inc. in Canada. This book truly reflects her dedication to helping others help themselves with TRT® as an invaluable complement to other methods of care through Hospice.

We have had the opportunity to read her manuscript, and we have been touched deeply by that experience. Now as you open your hearts to the experiences and sharings that unfold in this book, please take the moments to read deeply.

Thousands of students are using TRT®, a living science of energy that has been kept intact for you and others to study and to use in your daily life. Many students and Authorized Instructors choose to serve others with TRT®. We are celebrating the publication of *We Are Timeless: The Radiance Technique® in Hospice Care* and the companion DVD, which can open the way for more and more people around the world to serve the expansion of themselves and others with The Radiance Technique®.

~ Dr. Barbara Ray, Marvelle Lightfields, and Fred W. Wright Jr.

When I first studied The Radiance Technique®,
I thought I was going to learn something that
would help me recover from cancer
and help me with my physical health.
What I discovered is a rare jewel,
a way to support my whole self,
not only my body or mind.

~ *Christine Maria Gross*

Introduction

I sat beside Ralph's hospital bed as he moved into a coma, nearing his transition. Music played softly in the background and as I gently placed my hands over his heart, his face became serene, his breathing became more calm and even. A profound peace permeated the room.

I sensed from the interior of the living system of energy that we shared that all was radiantly alive and well. The room expanded: I was experiencing an opening above us, around us, and we were in the centre. Breath by breath, there was a deep sacredness in this silence. I was moving with him in an indescribable space of love, an ever-present reality. In the early hours, Ralph made his transition in Light.

Experiences such as this have led me to discover that there is more to life than death, more to death than our bodies. There is energy, a life force, which extends beyond our physical body and survives beyond our physical death. It has been known by many wise beings in diverse cultures throughout millennia. These wise ones remind us that we do not really die; we are eternal, immortal and infinite.

Within the pages of this book are people's direct experiences that go beyond the ordinary ways of viewing illness, death and dying using The Radiance Technique®, an ancient science of Universal Radiant Energy.

As used throughout this book, Radiant Energy is defined as follows:

Radiance, Radiant Energy — *Is Inner, Transcendental, Universal Light transmitted from within to the outer planes; the quality of luminosity; radiating Inner Light; emitting brilliant rays of shining, glowing Radiance. The Radiance Technique® accesses your Inner Radiance and expands upon this point of Inner Light without limit, Always in a never-ending Journey of healing/wholing, natural opening and growth, transformation and ultimately your Cosmic Birthright — Enlightenment.*[1]

The Radiance Technique® is a unique, ancient transcendental energy technique that has inner keys to support one in this life and beyond. It allows individuals to discover for themselves wisdom and truths known for thousands of years. Van Ault, a teacher of The Radiance Technique® who lived for many years with the AIDS virus, describes the technique this way:

> The Radiance Technique® is a whole and complete system for activating, restoring and balancing energy from within the individual. The system accesses a kind of energy present in all living things, but that is far beyond the mind, emotions, and physical senses. This kind of energy is referred to as _transcendental_, or _radiant_, and with TRT®, it can be generated through the hands and directed to oneself or others through the simple act of touch. The act of applying the energy in such a way is referred to here as _Radiant Touch®_ or _hands-on_. Additionally, the energy can be directed in ways without touch, which include what is called _distance directing or attunements_.[2]

The origins of The Radiance Technique® can be traced back to cultures such as Tibet and Egypt. TRT® is related to other Eastern vibrational sciences, including various kinds of transcendental meditations such as TM™, the Vedas, and authentic vibrational systems of mantra, mandala, and raja yoga. TRT® is an ancient knowledge revealing ways to access higher levels or frequencies of energy. Today, this method is readily accessible by anyone through an Authorized Instructor (See Appendices) and has been widely taught around the world since the 1970s. Its applications are vast, ranging from a technique for relaxation and quieting the mind to many ways for supporting someone in their dying process.

The Radiance Technique® has maintained an unbroken, intact development through thousands of years of history.

Dr. Barbara Ray, Ph.D., is the living authority on the authentic system of seven degrees within TRT®. Her academic background, specializing in classical civilizations and languages including studies of ancient Egypt and Near Eastern civilizations, enabled her to recognize TRT® and share the information with others who might have not studied humankind's past in such detail. She put this information into a contemporary perspective and made it accessible for modern times. There is a body of knowledge about TRT® available in Dr. Barbara Ray's books, including *The 'Reiki' Factor in The Radiance Technique®; The Expanded Reference Manual of The Radiance Technique®, Authentic Reiki®; The Official Handbook of The Radiance Technique®, Authentic Reiki®,* and *The Radiance Technique® and Managing Stress.*

The origins of TRT® in my life trace back to my own life-threatening illness. When I was first referred to hospice, I never heard about hospice or even knew what it meant. Like most 23-year-olds, I was focused on my future, finishing school and having a social life. But somewhere in the cards, there was a different path for me to take, and in 1988, my diagnosis with an advanced cancer began a life-changing direction for me.

As I was pushed off the diving board into the deep end, I found myself experiencing uncertainty, and I treaded water in the unknown. Nothing was familiar, and nothing was the same. I was plagued by fear, which made the process of recovery seem that much more daunting.

Joseph Chilton Pearce, biologist, researcher and author of *The Biology of Transcendence: A Blueprint of the Human Spirit*, writes, "Fear of death locks our mind into survival strategies that counter our discovery of possibilities other than death."

It was difficult for me to comprehend that my illness could supply any discoveries or possibilities that would be beneficial to me. I felt fragile and sensitive to inner and outer environments, and at the same time, I knew that something was sustaining me. Yes, my physical body was deteriorating and dying, but what was happening to the rest of me? What was the rest of me? Slowly, I realized I would have to take an active role in my recovery. I had to dig deep and search within myself for strength and answers. When I took responsibility for my health and well-being, I began learning more about myself. Through my prayers and meditations, I began to discover the possibilities for wholeness in my life.

I opened myself to a completely new way of perceiving. In exploring my dying, I discovered living. My journey was not about illness. It was about connecting with something vaster and greater. I became aware that I was a remarkable being made up of both physical and non-physical energy.

This awareness propelled me on a path of exploration with the healing arts, contemplative religions, practices, and native healing methods. I read various texts, attended spiritual gatherings, travelled and met wonderful teachers, guides, mentors and healers. I embraced many complementary and alternative therapies before, during and after my diagnosis. Classical healing systems of Ayurveda, Traditional Chinese and Tibetan medical traditions became partners in my care plan. Each has an entirely different approach to disease than Western allopathic medicine and offers much wisdom. Although I recognized the benefits of the allopathic treatments that I received, it was clear that our traditional medical system had limitations. So I utilized the best of both worlds and married the western and eastern philosophies.

Then I met with The Radiance Technique® and a whole new dimension unfolded. When I first studied TRT®, I thought I was going to learn something that would help me recover from cancer and help me with my physical health. What I discovered is a rare jewel, a way to support my whole self, not only my body or mind. It was different from my other meditations because I would use my hands on specific areas on my body. A form of transcendental meditation, my TRT® hands-on meditations facilitated deep relaxation, increased energy, and vitality within me.

I learned a complete energy balancing procedure in which my hands direct energy to 12 positions on my body, beginning at my head and ending at the base of my spine. TRT® opened the door of real learning and discovery through my own experiences. I certainly did not know that much about TRT® when I took my first course, like how and why it worked, but it did not stop me from using it or receiving its benefits. This is not unusual; I interact and use different types of energy all the time, unaware of the mechanics. One example, when I turn on the ignition, I know that my car runs as long as I filled up the gas tank, but I don't know any intricate details why it works, and I can still use my car. It is the same with TRT®. I do not need to be especially gifted or have special knowledge or believe in it to use it.

TRT® goes beyond stress management to restoring and retaining energy on all levels. I realized that things I did each day did not regenerate me, and like many people today, I often lived with an energy deficit. Filling up my reservoir daily with whole, balancing energy made a lot of sense to me. As TRT® restored energy to my whole body-mind-emotion-spirit dynamic, gentle shifts took place within me. I became more perceptive of my physical being, of where I held stress and of how I reacted to stress and when I felt depleted. I saw myself as a walking laboratory in which I could observe myself and get direct feedback of my biological interactions with the Radiant light energy.

The relaxation of my parasympathetic nervous system was producing calmness and deep rest throughout my whole body. The increasing circulation to my body's organs brought more colour to my complexion. I looked forward to my daily hour of meditation and increased the time as needed. On days when I missed a session, I definitely felt a difference in how I managed my day and reacted to events around me.

When faced with stressful situations, I immediately utilized shorter moments of hands-on positions and it supported me in responding. The simplicity of this form of Radiant Touch® differentiates TRT® from other energy methods and meditation techniques. I could practice it anywhere at any time and was not confined to closing my eyes. I could even use it while waiting for appointments, driving, watching television or reading a book.

The TRT® sessions released calming neurotransmitters and hormones to my endocrine system. I observed that as my body relaxed, my mind responded to the Radiant energy. The one hour spent in hands-on meditation supported me to just "be" with my busy thoughts and provided the time to download and let go. My mind was like my computer. With too much information, my computer crashed. As I continued my sessions, I realized the value such a practice had on my thoughts. My mind became clearer and less cluttered, and my memory improved. The sessions effortlessly released my stress and guided me into deeper realizations of peace.

I found relief in the fact that I did not need my mind to make the Radiant energy flow. My teacher assured me that once the initiatory attunement processes were activated within me, the transcendental nature of this energy system would naturally bypass the mind. Accessing the energy was not limited by whether I could concentrate or keep my mind steady. So in placing my hands on the specific positions I was taught, nothing could affect the energy I was accessing. I did not have to be in or create the "right" frame of mind to connect. I did not need to visualize, recite, repeat words or even concentrate. I did not have to go into an altered state. Its effectiveness was not dependent on my state of awareness. It was so simple. I was even able to use it when I was feeling tired. This transcendental energy technique was beyond thought. In transcending, my mind was settling inward to my innermost self, providing me with deep peace and restfulness. I realized what a great advantage this technique offered for those unable to focus.

TRT® provided an opportunity to serve in a profound way, and I grew in my understanding and experience of the immense capacity of the energy of The Radiance Technique® when I began supporting others through hospice. The hospice movement has uncovered and recovered dignity regarding dying and supports one's capacity to face death in our death phobic society. From my own experiences, I realized how TRT® could help others find peace amid the chaos that illness often creates. I volunteered as newsletter editor with Hospice after my chemotherapy treatments. A year later, I returned to introduce TRT® hands-on sessions to staff and management as a supportive method for patients. One by one, mini sessions were given, and relaxation by staff ensued.

Convinced of the technique's benefits for hospice clients, The Hospice of Windsor and Essex County Inc. established a Radiant Touch® Program in 1992. Through the Day Hospice, I began offering sessions along with a colleague. We provided this service to patients and their caregivers to support a better quality of life.

I realized that my ongoing practice of TRT® was not just for my benefit but also for the benefit of others. It became clear that I wanted to teach others this method and five years after learning TRT®, I became an Authorized Instructor. This greatly expanded my ability to help others and equipped me with additional techniques to support the healing/wholing♥ process. As the well-known Chinese proverb says, "*If you give a man a fish, he will eat for a day. If you teach a man how to fish, he will eat for a lifetime.*" When students have completed study of The First Degree Official Program of The Radiance Technique®, they will then have Radiant Touch®.

A remarkable realization is how TRT® has deepened my capacity for compassion and unconditional love and diminished my idea of separateness of self. The purpose of TRT® is to expand "Real Light."♥♥ I am Light and this journey is one of becoming conscious of these inner dimensions. As I continue, I experience an incredible healing in touching and recognizing this sacred light within everyone. In extending my hands to others, I am reminded of my own mortality, and through TRT®, I embrace my eternal self. So much of this is an inward journey, without form or words and beyond what I am able to perceive and communicate. The Radiance Technique®, for me, is living an ordinary life in an extraordinary way.

TRT® has made a significant and profound contribution to those involved in hospice care. *We Are Timeless: The Radiance Technique® in Hospice Care* is an attempt to document that contribution. It explores how individuals can live more fully here now despite the stress surrounding illness and how TRT® balances, transforms and enlightens bodies, minds and emotions of both those needing care and caregivers. The content in these pages tell how TRT® supports people in all stages of life, recording how they discover possibilities of well-being and greater quality of life, no matter what is happening physically.

The candid sharings of the contributors show how generating Radiant energy supports professionals and volunteers caring for the sick, sustains caregivers and comforts, guides and inspires people coping with illness and those moving through the dying process. The personal stories and anecdotes illuminate questions about life and death, supporting an expanding awareness of the infinite energy within.

For me, the experience of interacting, collecting and meditating with each sharing has brought transformation and change. The compassion and love expressed in these pages continue to touch me daily.

Combining The Radiance Technique® with hospice care has given me an amazing opportunity to discover how life can be lived fully in the here now, whether driving to work, writing a report, attending meetings, eating lunch, talking to families, or visiting a dying person. It connects me to a deeper understanding of compassion and allows me to recognize that my life can be one of service from a point of love.

TRT® is practised all over the world and has been integrated into health care centres and facilities such as The Hospice of Windsor and Essex County Inc., the oldest and largest community-based hospice in Canada where I have been working for 20 years offering a Radiant Touch® program with a dedicated group of volunteers.

As I complete this book, which has been a worldwide community effort, the season of spring greets me with renewal and celebration. It has been 20 years since I first studied The Radiance Technique®, and I am thankful for it every day of my life.

With deep gratitude, I honour everyone who contributed to the writing and recording of the many experiences shared. I hold within my heart a joyful reverence to all as we journey together in Light.

~ Christine Maria Gross

---

¹ Barbara Ray, Ph.D., *The Expanded Reference Manual of The Radiance Technique®, Authentic Reiki®,* (St. Petersburg, FL: Radiance Associates, 1987), p. 91.

² Van Ault, *The Radiance Technique® and AIDS,* (San Francisco, CA: Resources for Renewal, 1996), p. 1.

³ Joseph Chilton Pearce, *The Biology of Transcendence. A Blueprint of the Human Spirit,* (Rochester, Vermont: Inner Traditions International, 2002), p. 235.

♥As Dr. Barbara Ray writes in *The Expanded Reference Manual of The Radiance®, Authentic Reiki®* about healing:

Healing/Wholing - The verb 'to heal' derives from an Old English root meaning 'to make whole.' The Radiance Technique® accesses an energy which is *whole* and which in an unfolding process interacts with other, not whole, not universal energies in such a way as to move in the direction of wholeness. 'Healing' in its true and simple meaning refers to a process of 'wholing.' In this context, The Radiance Technique® is a science of universal energy promoting the healing/wholing process. Medical healing is different from and in no way connected to The Radiance Technique®, its techniques and its processes. The Radiance Technique® has *nothing whatever* to do with any form of 'practicing medicine,' or prescribing drugs or of diagnosing. The Radiance Technique® is *not* a science of disease — it is a science of universal energy and of wholeness.

Barbara Ray, Ph.D., *The Expanded Reference Manual of The Radiance Technique®, Authentic Reiki®*, (St. Petersburg, FL: Radiance Associates, 1987), p. 50.

♥♥ Real Light is not sensational to the outer senses and TRT® accesses this higher vibration of unlimited, eternal light. As Dr. Barbara Ray writes,

Light -There is light in the physical sense which can be seen by the outer, physical eye. Kinds of natural, physical light include sunlight and its reflections, and electrical light, lightning, and there are kinds of artificial light. There is also a kind of *Light* which can only be seen by the inner eye and is not visible to the outer physical eye called Transcendental, Universal *Light*. It is this Inner, Transcendental Light-energy which is accessed directly through the inner dynamic of the intact science of The Radiance Technique®..."

Ibid., p. 66.

PART 1

At the centre of all love I stand,
and naught can touch me here,
and from that centre
I shall go forth to love and serve.

~ Alice A. Bailey

Compassionate Touch
in Hospice Care

*The Radiance Technique® supports
our patients in the final stages of their lives
creating a peaceful and calming transition.
TRT® is an excellent support for
patients and families to draw
on during any stage of the
disease process and we
are grateful to have
it available.*

*~ Carol Derbyshire
Executive Director
The Hospice of Windsor and Essex County Inc.*

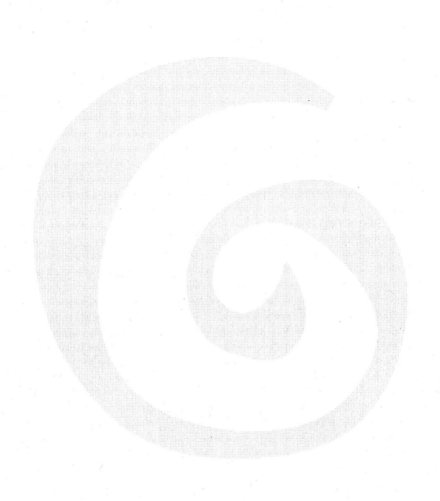

-1-

THE VERY NATURE OF HOSPICE IS COMPASSION. "Cum passion" in Latin means "with suffering." In the fourth century, the hospice began as a refuge for travelers on a difficult journey. It was a place where pilgrims came to be healed when cure was no longer possible. A place of comfort, love and caring. A place of relief, not pain. Compassion is the gift of being with one who is suffering, and one of the qualities of The Radiance Technique® is the principle of universal love. "From the energies of universal love comes the energy of Compassion."[1]

Today, hospice describes both a concept and a program of support known as palliative care. British physician Dame Cicely Saunders and American physician Dr. Elisabeth Kübler-Ross were two pioneers of the modern hospice movement. According to The Canadian Hospice Palliative Care Association, "Hospice palliative care aims to relieve suffering and improve the quality of living and dying."[2]

The Hospice of Windsor and Essex County Inc.

The Hospice that provided care to me has expanded and redefined itself over the years. In the spring of 1992, The Hospice of Windsor and Essex County embarked on a new concept and created a Wellness Centre to support patients and caregivers. It already had been serving the community since 1979, and the "Day Hospice" was the first of its kind in Canada modeled after the British Hospice day away program for patients. Hospice professionals saw that disease not only affects patients, but also their families and caregivers. The mission of Hospice is to *support, educate and empower those who are affected by or caring for a person with a life-altering diagnosis in order to achieve their desired quality of life.*

This unique approach, to support people at the beginning of their diagnosis, not just in their last few months, pushed our Hospice beyond the boundaries of traditional hospice care. The concept of care at any stage of the disease spectrum was new; no one else in North America was doing it. Earlier hospice care can have a positive effect on the quality of life of both patients and their caregivers. Helping people get on with their living, helping them feel they are not alone and empowering individuals at any stage in their illness process are the focus of the Hospice's unique programs and supportive care services.

Hospice did not fit the mould of most of Canada in its progressive ideas nor in its caseload. Serving over 800 families in 2011, it is the oldest and largest palliative care facility in Canada. Beyond numbers, what sets this Hospice apart from others is the ability to mobilize partnerships with local hospitals, health councils and public education facilities to assure continuity of care. For over 30 years, Windsor Hospice has kept palliative care on the local, provincial and national agenda and in the minds and hearts of many.

Hospice has evolved dramatically and on April 16, 2007, over five hundred community supporters, local officials, MPPs, along with the Minister of Health, George Smitherman, celebrated the opening of an eight bed residential home facility at Canada's first Hospice Village. Currently, Hospice has an interdisciplinary team of 44 staff consisting of social workers, nurses, physicians, program coordinators, administrative and fundraising staff along with over 750 volunteers. Each team member plays a vital role and brings unique skills to contribute to high quality care. The high numbers of new diagnosis are indicative of the trend of an aging population, but more shockingly is that Windsor and its surrounding area, with a total population of 393,402[3] has the highest levels of cancer, cardiovascular and lung related diseases in all of Canada.[4] Cancer Care Ontario has regional cancer programs and studies continuing to address the increasing numbers, and several other provincial cities share Windsor's high cancer rates.

Yet, despite efforts, the numbers of people with illness continue to rise. Hospice provides resources to access information, education, peer support and professional support, and all of these services are free of charge. These services focus on comfort measures, emotional and spiritual support, pain and symptom management, and respite and grief support for caregivers. And so when the Wellness Centre blossomed in the spring of 1992, the gentle touch of The Radiance Technique® became an integral part of the Centre's programming along with standard levels of care and treatment. The Ontario Ministry of Health, Long-Term Care Branch provided funding for the program.

TRT® in Hospice Care

"Hospices were founded on the principle of helping people who are dying to live as fully as possible, and TRT®, with its life-enhancing and wholing qualities, combines naturally with all aspects of hospice care," says British Hospice social worker, Maya Melrose.

The Radiance Technique® is accepted in hospices, hospitals, cancer centres, AIDS centres and long-term care facilities because it is effective in promoting relaxation, reducing pain and lowering anxiety levels. This technique helps patients and caregivers by releasing stress that, in turn, can help them in their recovery and treatment. TRT® also comforts, supports and eases the dying process.

Over the past 20 years, executive director Carol Derbyshire has worked tirelessly to create a community Hospice in Windsor and Essex County. She is a visionary in her field. Carol is recognized and respected as a leader in palliative care and has rallied with the board of directors to bring many medical services and innovative programs to the community, including TRT®.

Carol champions the value of TRT® at Hospice. "The Radiance Technique® has touched the lives of many of our patients and family members here at The Hospice of Windsor and Essex County," she observes. "We have been offering TRT® since 1992, and I can honestly say that it is one of the most popular programs — thousands of people have benefitted from it. Last year, volunteers gave over 2,000 hours of hands-on sessions.

"Often patients call us having just received news of a diagnosis. They are frightened, anxious and unable to think clearly. After a session of Radiant Touch® with one of our volunteer practitioners or staff, patients feel a sense of control again and are able to begin to work through the chaos that this diagnosis often creates.

"We encourage people to complete four sessions of Radiant Touch®, and we find that people are feeling more peaceful deep within themselves. Their anxiety lessens, and they are better able to cope with their illness. It is a wonderful beginning point to support people in reaching a feeling of empowerment and openness to accept further support. Patients and their caregivers also have the opportunity to learn this technique in a certified training that we offer as well.

"The Radiance Technique® also supports our patients in the final stages of their lives, creating a peaceful and calming transition. TRT® is an excellent support for patients and families to draw on during any stage of the disease process, and we are grateful to have it available."

Referral Process

Patients and family members can refer themselves for sessions of Radiant Touch®. Professionals from the Community Care Access Centre, the Windsor Regional Cancer Centre, local hospitals, clinics, and long-term care facilities also refer clients to the program.

Radiant Touch® is available to patients, their caregivers, partners and support persons. As well, volunteers, staff and professional caregivers may access the service. TRT® can assist in many ways.

Benefits of The Radiance Technique®
- release stress and anxiety
- relax and quiet the mind
- calm and soothe the emotions
- improve sense of well-being
- promotion of sleep and deep rest
- natural pain release and change in perception of pain
- restore and balance natural flow of life force energy
- spiritual support
- comfort
- enhance quality of life
- connect to inner stillness
- energy support for a peaceful transition

Radiant Touch® at Cancer Centre

In fall 2001, in partnership with the Windsor Regional Cancer Centre, Hospice began to offer Radiant Touch® on site to patients during chemotherapy treatments and before or after medical procedures. There is a special room in the

Supportive Care wing where hospice volunteers provide sessions to patients and their caregivers.

Oncologist Dr. Hakam Abu-Zahra recommends TRT® to patients and says in an interview, "The Radiance Technique® is of great benefit to any person but especially to those patients in need of palliative care. I am talking about patients who have had recurrence of their cancer and as a result are suffering from its complications — for example, having pain, extreme anxiety or lack of sleep. I found that The Radiance Technique® is very helpful in alleviating these symptoms and supporting a better quality of life for many of these patients."

The Radiance Technique® Stages of Supportive Care:
- pre-diagnosis and diagnosis
- pre and post surgery, post operative relaxation
- coping with illness
- chemotherapy, radiation, other medical procedures
- wellness (post-treatment, post-cancer, other)
- recurrence of disease
- dying process
- coping-caregiver relief, stress relief
- crisis
- grieving/bereavement

Healing Touch

You may be wondering how a technique can support so many different aspects of a person. Mentioned earlier, TRT® is a technique to support the *whole* person. This means that the energy within TRT® supports all the different parts of ourselves that make up who we are. Beginning at the centre of our consciousness, our innermost selves, the energy of TRT® ripples out balancing our physical, mental and emotional levels.

Within our western (allopathic) traditional medical model, the focus of healing has been on the physical with little focus on other dimensions of us. Particularly in hospice care, we are beginning to acknowledge the many dimensions that contribute to our healing. These many dimensions make up our energy system.

Radiant Touch® Supports Medical Care Practices

Touch is multi-dimensional. The way we are touched physically affects us on many levels. Patients are still often touched in an objective scientific manner. Being poked for blood, palpitated for lumps, radiated for tumours, scanned and x-rayed for abnormalities and cut open to remove growths, must be done with sensitivity. Otherwise, a lack of compassion increases the alienation a person already feels for him/herself and lack of connection to his/her body. Dr. Barbara Ray shares, *The mechanistic approach is not wrong in that it recognizes a need to treat an injured or diseased physical part; but it tends to exclude the greater truth that all parts of your being must be activated in the healing process. ...*[5]

TRT® can support medical care practices such as chemotherapy, radiation and drug therapies. Any medical procedure can be enhanced naturally with The Radiance Technique®, and every touch related contact becomes an opportunity for the vibration of universal love to be expressed. A Radiant hand on the heart centre to assist in relaxing the breath, over the vein that was injected with chemotherapy, on the head area to assist in calming during a painful bone marrow procedure are a few examples of the complementary, nurturing nature of TRT®.

June James R.N., a former nurse educator with Hospice, shares an experience using TRT® during chemotherapy:

"Ann, a 45-year-old professional woman recently diagnosed with advanced cancer of the ovary, was admitted to the hospital to start chemotherapy. During my initial intervention, the chemotherapy nurse came in to start her IV. Immediately, Ann became extremely anxious, upset and tearful and spoke of her intense phobia about needles and injections. I asked her if I could do a relaxation technique using my hands, and she agreed.

"When I placed my hands in Front Position #1, I could feel her racing heart. Within a minute, I could feel her heartbeat return to normal, and the venepuncture procedure was completed quickly and successfully. I continued TRT® for about 20 minutes, and when finished, she expressed her gratitude by telling me, 'That was paradise.' This intervention led to a very positive initiation of treatment for her and decreased her emotional pain and anxiety tremendously."

From the moment June placed her hands on Ann's body, there was an instantaneous connection to Radiant energy taking place. This happens because June's hands were activated in The First Degree Official Program of The Radiance Technique®, Authentic Reiki® seminar so that transcendental energy is always present every time she touches.

The key role of the practitioner is to *share* a session, for support, balance and harmony. Universal energy travels to wherever the receiver needs it. June's sharing illustrates a physical, mental and emotional interaction Ann had with the Radiant energy. A session re-establishes the natural rhythm and flow of energy. Whatever one experiences will be uniquely one's own. Both the giver and receiver benefit. Dr. Barbara Ray writes:

> **Receiver** - *When using The Radiance Technique®, the receiver, to whom the universal Radiance is directed, whether it is yourself, others, animals, plants or whatever, receives according to his/her <u>inner</u> needs radiating from within to without. The person transmitting cannot control, manipulate or interfere with the Radiant Wholeness of universal energy and cannot <u>harm</u> another with this kind of energy.*[6]

A Unique Kind of Balancing Technique

TRT® is different from most energy techniques we are familiar with in that *TRT® is not about doing something to someone.*
Diagnosing, scanning, or intent to make something happen
are not involved in the process. TRT® is neither a channelling
nor a drawing out of energy technique. It is not about sens-
ing or having physical sensations nor visualizing or producing
certain feelings. The mind and emotions are not involved in
accessing the energy of TRT®, because it naturally bypasses
the mind and personality. The ease and use of TRT® provides
a way to balance ourselves on all levels and opens to us an
actual vibration of wholeness that we can experience.

A Typical TRT® Session

Since TRT® requires no special equipment, it can be provided
virtually anywhere, anytime. A typical session lasts one hour
and can be shorter, depending on the need or situation. TRT®
does not require the formal 12-position session for the giver
to transmit energy to the receiver as demonstrated in the previous sharing from June.

During a session, people rest fully clothed wherever
they are. This could be while in a chair or even standing up.
Sessions can also take place on a comfortable massage table,
in a recliner chair, on a sofa, in a wheelchair or while lying in
bed. Relaxing music may be played softly in the background
to support a healing environment.

It is not necessary to physically touch the body during a
session. Hands can be held eight to ten centimetres above the
body, and in cases where practitioners have taken advanced
training in techniques like *directing*, they do not need to have
their hands physically near the body. Most of the time people
feel comfortable with the feather-light touch TRT® offers.
This contact is often the only contact people receive in their

day or week. I will never forget the words expressed by one patient to me, "I am so glad that you are not afraid to touch my body."

In a basic hands-on session, the practitioner places his or her hands on or above 12 areas of the body. Each hand position is held for approximately five minutes. These areas are not random, but follow a specific sequence on the body. First beginning at the head and ending at the base of the spine. Throughout the book, they will be written as *Head Positions #1-4, Front Positions #1-4, and Back Positions #1-4*. The locations of these positions correspond to the *seven major energy centres* or *chakras*.

These centres are unseen, invisible, energy vortices in constant movement all the time with no physical location. They are transformers of energy that have natural locations within the body and interact with our outer bodies. Most people only know these three levels of consciousness or outer bodies: body, emotions and mind. But there is a higher nature of reality known as transcendental. In Vedic Medicine, the understanding is that we, as human beings, are really an energetic system organized around different layers of consciousness known as *subtle bodies*. (See Energy Model used in TRT®in Appendices) TRT®is a science of healing that accesses these multi-dimensional chakras to allow the individual to access different experiences and states of consciousness. Hands-on or directing with the chakras generate, balance and restore vital energy to the various bodies of an individual.

TRT®can be used in many ways. Many people use it as meditation. Others use TRT®as a form of bodywork, a healing technique that many say is effective in promoting well-being and coping with physical ailments. People's experiences with TRT®vary from physical to spiritual, from tangible to intangible. The full affects of TRT® may never be fully known, nor can they yet be empirically measured.

Currently at Hospice, nurses, social workers and a team

of volunteers provide TRT®in a variety of settings. They include homes, hospitals, and long-term care facilities as well as the Hospice Wellness Centre and Residential Homes, and onsite at the Windsor Regional Cancer Centre. Members of the Radiant Touch® volunteer team who have shared their experiences here have responded from within, and their work through Hospice is a gesture of service to fellow human beings in time of need.

[1] Barbara Ray, Ph.D., *The Expanded Reference Manual of The Radiance Technique®, Authentic Reiki®,* (St. Petersburg, FL: Radiance Associates, 1987), p. 113.

[2] Canadian Hospice Palliative Care Association, *A Model to Guide Hospice Palliative Care,* (Ottawa, ON: CHPCA, 2002), p. 17.

[3] StatisticsCensus Canada, 2006 Census www.statcan.ca.

[4] Community Health Profile of Windsor, Ontario, Canada: Anatomy of a Great Lakes Area of Concern, Michael Gilbertson and James Brophy, International Joint Commission, *Environmental Health Perspectives Volume 109, Supplement 6, December 2001.*

[5] Barbara Ray, Ph.D., *The 'Reiki' Factor in The Radiance Technique® Expanded Edition,* (St. Petersburg, FL: Radiance Associates, 1992), p. 15.

[6] Ray, *The Expanded Reference Manual of The Radiance Technique®, Authentic Reiki®,* p. 92.

May the love we're sharing spread its wings
And fly across the earth
And bring new joy to every soul who is alive.
May the blessings of your grace my love
Shine on everyone and may we all see the Light
Within, within, within.

~ Traditional Song

Volunteering from the Heart

*At the age of 70, I now have a
deeper understanding of caregiving,
and my capacity for being with
patients has expanded.
During TRT® hands-on or
directing, there is an unspoken
communication and connection.*

*Rita Lepp
Hospice Radiant Touch® Volunteer*

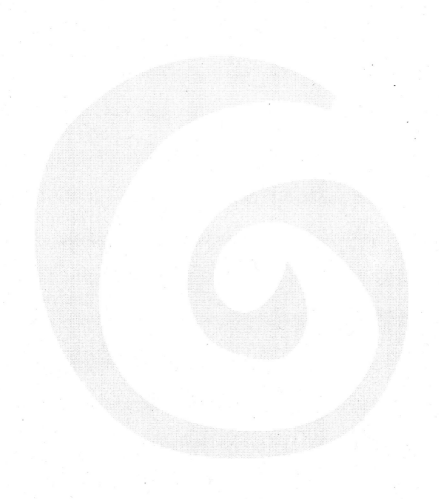

-2-

D EMONSTRATING THE BASIC UNIVERSAL HUMAN qualities of care, love, compassion and concern for the welfare of
others, volunteers make the world a better place for us to live
in, and to die in. This truly is service from the heart. As Dr.
Barbara Ray says, "A profound and true Healing/Wholing
begins within you when you dedicate and give selflessly,
Service to something larger than yourself."[1]

The key to our own well-being is inherently connected to
our love and care for our fellow human beings. Volunteers are
the heart and soul of Hospice and the Radiant Touch® team.
All ages and all walks of life make up this dedicated group of
volunteers. The spirit has emerged in many ordinary people
who heard a call from within and provide countless hours of
service to many.

Some people volunteer because they want to give back
to society. Others share their time to return the support they
personally received. Each one has a story of someone in the
family, a friend, a colleague or a neighbour who experienced a
serious illness and/or death. They feel blessed to be alive and
want to help others in their time of need. Many wish
to continue their nurturing roles, and Joan Caba is one such
volunteer.

"As a registered nurse, I have always enjoyed helping
people," says Joan. "Now that I have retired, my experience
helps me understand the physiological changes my clients are
experiencing. With TRT®, it is an honour to be a comfort to a
client and the family when death is near. I feel it is a privilege

to be with people as they go through their personal journey at this very important time of their lives. Nothing superficial... no time for that... just honest feelings and caring for each other. My patients are most appreciative of the time we spend together, and I receive so much from being with them."

Volunteer Training

Volunteers for each area of Hospice complete the required 36-hour patient care training that complies with the Hospice Association of Ontario Standards of Practice and have at least one-year of experience with patients before training for Radiant Touch®.

There are two components of the Radiant Touch® volunteer training program. *The First Degree Official Program of The Radiance Technique®, Authentic Reiki®* the initial level, consists of a 12-hour seminar with an Authorized Instructor credentialed through the certifying body: Radiance Seminars, Inc. This corporation develops the training and sets the professional standards and ethical principles for Authorized Instructors worldwide.

The second component involves a specialized course, *Hospice Care Practitioner Training in Radiant Touch®*. This training was developed with input from patients, caregivers and volunteers. It includes 35 hours of class time and 120 hours of hands-on experience, case studies, reading and self-care. It is an intensive course, but when volunteers complete it, they always say that they want more. In response to this request, we provide ongoing support throughout the year in a variety of ways.

Radiant Touch® Support Groups

"Support nights" provide the opportunity for volunteers to share stories, experiences, songs, tears, laughter and home-made cookies. We also offer group marathon sessions, which are another way to amplify energy and provide support through receiving two hours or more of non-stop Radiant energy.

Throughout the year, continuing education and "expansion classes" offer volunteers the opportunity to deepen their use of TRT® for themselves as well as their patients. We also incorporate special theme nights facilitated by one of the volunteers. Such evenings have included exploring The Radiance Technique® with yoga, dance, chanting, painting, weaving and walking the labyrinth.

John Bondy documents many of our radiant events. He enjoys photography and is a member of the Hospice Volunteer Advisory Board. John has The Second Degree and finds benefit in the TRT® support activities for volunteers: "My quality of life has improved dramatically with TRT® marathons and with our Radiant Touch® support group. It is essential to me to share ideas and experiences, personal growth, Radiant energy, hugs, laughter, and to share common ground and feelings about our Hospice patients we care for and to honour their passing. I feel the love I have experienced and shared has expanded the love I have for people. I feel closer to people at work and in the community I previously would not have felt close to."

Pat Bachand, another volunteer, finds that, "when we get together with our radiant group, it is our family... like a home coming."

Group Exchanges

The Hospice volunteer team meets monthly for group hands-on exchanges as a time of support to each other. Volunteers gather around massage tables in groups of three or more. Each volunteer receives a turn to be a recipient on the table. It is a different experience than being just with one practitioner, as a session can be given in a shorter period. As well, each pair of Radiant hands expands the total energy exponentially, and many comment on the energy boosting and healing qualities of the group energy.

One volunteer on the receiving end of a group exchange experienced a powerful healing on several levels:

"The night we met, I had a headache that was into its second week and I was into my fourth week of having no feelings in my legs or feet. Halfway through the hands-on session, I actually began to experience feeling in my legs and before I knew my headache was gone. I felt like I was floating free from pain and filled with light and love. I never in my life expected such a healing to occur," recalls Rosemary McGregor.

"I found this encounter very spiritual, and as tears rolled down my cheeks, I knew how blessed and how touched I was by this experience. Now I know how my patients at Hospice feel. I always knew TRT® made a positive change for them, but never to what degree. I thank God for this technique. You see, I believe my illness gave me the opportunity to experience a healing from TRT®. Now I know what it is to receive and I have a deeper appreciation of how important my service in Radiant Touch® is to Hospice."

John Brownlie, a Naturalist at Point Pelee National Park, recalling his very first radiant group exchange, noticed a shift in perception simply by changing focus: "I'll always remember the first time I listened with my hands," he says. "I had just completed my training and joined the Radiant Touch® volunteer team. We were sharing a group hands-on session for one of the members. During the session, Christine encouraged us to listen with our hands. Wow! What a difference! I could feel a shift as the members changed their focus to listening. I remember being very impressed with this and I use this listening approach when doing hands-on with patients."

The self-help component of the hospice training is a vital aspect, and volunteers like Sherry Brunelle state their surprise at its inclusion in the program. She wanted to learn TRT® to help her patients, but found out that it would help her, too.

"At first I admit I was disappointed, because I wanted to learn TRT®for my patients, and my teacher said the first part was to focus on ourselves. Self-healing was the order of the day. It was hard for me at first to think of me," confides Sherry. "I was always doing for others, and here I wanted to do a technique for others. However, it did not take me long to realize that it was exactly what I really needed. The reservoir concept of restoring depleted energy to me was the convincing part for me to do TRT®."

Volunteer Care

TRT® for Self-Help

As Sherry discovered, The Radiance Technique®'s restorative qualities are a real bonus for volunteers. Care for the volunteer is essential and enables the volunteer to be more relaxed, peaceful and present with their patients. Applying this method of natural healing on a daily basis strengthens the ability to take in vital life energy.

Healing can happen on many levels. TRT® provides Sherry with physical and mental relief. "I have fibromyalgia and before studying TRT®, I was taking many medications for my pain," she recounts. "I used to get many headaches and many body aches, and I was not able to focus on many things. Poor memory was another symptom. I must say that I use my pain medications very little now. When headaches or head pain come, I do the first four Head Positions and most of the pain goes away. Being able to focus on and accomplish projects, has, of course, made me a more relaxed and calmer person."

John Bondy has found that TRT® has made a difference in his quality of life: "The Radiance Technique® has shown me that I need to take time for myself away from the distractions of daily life," says John. "I have used TRT® to help me with chronic prostatitis and in balancing my health. It has not cured me, but it has helped me. I have found direct hands-on to an area hurting usually brings either full or partial relief. I use the full hands-on positions and also do a mini session before I go to work in the morning."

Another volunteer writes of the health benefits she receives from using TRT®. Rosanna Crognale has found it to be a great support in the past five years:

"I practice the one hour session on myself and on others, and, daily, I do mini 'stress buster' sessions on myself. I just feel so much better. I have been a heavy duty asthmatic for 22 years, relying on maximum doses of medications. Now I seldom have attacks and seldom take medication. I only have the telltale signs of asthma when I get a respiratory infection, maybe once a year now, down from the annual three.

"When I get frustrated or angry, I immediately receive a massive headache, with constant pounding pain, shutting my eyes. There is no better evidence of the mind, body, spirit, wholing connection of TRT® for me than what I have experienced. For me, TRT® is a wholing process connecting us as beings in direct communication with the world around us."

When Lori first experienced TRT®, it was when her mother was sick with cancer. During this difficult time, her sessions helped her cope, "It was as if a weight lifted away." Lori took the training to bring this relief to others.

"In the early stages of the training, we learned TRT® as a self-help technique, and I found it difficult to lie still for an hour and had to force myself to do it. Today, it is just the opposite. I look forward to my daily session and thoroughly enjoy this time for me! My personal sessions are up to one hour and twenty minutes. The most soothing for me are Front Positions #1-4. I have reaped the benefits through TRT® and a number of changes have occurred. I find that I have become more centred, and more balanced as opposed to being rushed. There is calmness present within me rather than stress. I feel a depth of peace that I cannot explain. I also noticed that pets are drawn to me when the session is in process.

"The next best thing to a Radiant Touch® session that we perform on ourselves is to have this performed by another person attuned to TRT®. I experience the energy deeper and stronger. Having another person share a session makes me feel secure, comforted and at peace. I can only describe it by comparing it to the comfort of a mother's love, and one great big hug; it's very nurturing."

TRT®'s nurturing capacities are also felt by Cheryl Thomson: "Since learning this self-help technique, I indulge myself daily. It seems like indulgence because I get so much out of it. A first instinct was 'this is too good to be true.' TRT® is such a simple non-invasive technique, yet it is so powerful and peaceful. In this workaholic, multitask-oriented society, it could be considered 'wasted time.' I now know better. However, a year ago, I could never have imagined sitting still, or laying down quiet for one hour each day. I would have said that I do not have the time. Now I make the time and it is the most important hour of my day. It is my internal hug. It is my soul's nourishment.

"I consider it my best gift to myself. The gift of silence. Solitude. Peace. Tranquility. Self-esteem. Confidence. Calmness. Beauty. Joy.

"I can almost feel a merging and mingling of all the essences of being on all the different levels. It is a coming together spiritually, mentally, emotionally and physically. Coming together sometimes in a quick tempo jig, other times at a slow mellow swaying and surging until all feels right. Radiance is the composer and choreographer of my dance of the day.

"I've come to know I have to be patient and let it be the leader. I just have to follow the lead presented. Allow the present to unfold, as it should, without my conscious effort to control, manipulate or try to set the future in the direction of my choice. This has been a major lesson for me.

"On days that I have a session scheduled I look forward to that time. It is amazing to me that both the person giving and the person receiving are affected. I really adhere to the expression that the universe will provide whatever is necessary for the highest good.

"The practice of TRT® on myself and on others has led me to a new place. A place that is much more comfortable for me. There is a new awareness. I feel more thankful and peaceful. I feel much more relaxed about accepting what the future holds and filled with gratitude, knowing that I have a companion I can count on."

Beyond the Senses

Cindy Robinet works for Family Respite Services as a counsellor helping children and their families in Windsor, and she volunteers on the weekend for Hospice. "Last year, I was part of a group learning all about universal, Radiant energy, how to access it, and apply it to myself and others. However, I must admit I was a bit skeptic," admits Cindy. "How could you access something you cannot see, smell, touch or taste? Either I believed in vibrational energy or all those patients at Met Hospital who told me how it helped them were delusional and grasping at straws. Frankly, I believe in people, and if they said TRT® helped them, then I believed them. After all, it was not too long ago the medical profession pooh-poohed hand-washing and sterilization practices. What I did not expect was the personal satisfaction I'd receive.

"To my surprise, I found The Radiance Technique® training classes a joy to attend. Here I was, surrounded by a group of volunteers who shared the same outlook on life as I did.

They were there for the same reasons I was: to learn and help others. By the end of a workday, I'd be tired and what I call 'people pooped.' I spend most of my working hours talking with and counselling families who are caring for children with disabilities. Although I love my job and wouldn't trade it for the world, by 6 p.m., I'm ready for a quiet evening of reading or weaving baskets. The last thing I want to do is go out and socialize. But as I said earlier, to my surprise, I found the training sessions a joy. After spending an evening learning and practicing TRT®, I felt more relaxed and in touch with God and the universe. Instead of being tired, I felt rested and for lack of a better expression, at peace.

"Even if I cannot see, feel, taste or touch the energy, I know it is there. God is energy and I cannot see, feel, taste or touch Him either. It's called faith and I believe I'm able to access and share some of his love through TRT®. Radiant Touch® is about sharing. Sharing an experience. Sharing love."

The Radiance Technique® has contributed to John Bondy's emotional well-being and his awareness about it. "TRT® has helped me handle emotions such as fear, anger and grief through opening myself to these emotions and exploring them," he explains. "Hands-on has helped me accept my feelings and transform them into more love for myself and others. TRT® has helped me to be more loving and accept myself more fully, both my weaknesses and strengths. I feel more caring towards others. I feel a greater love for my family, all nature and people. The love that I experience with TRT® permeates my whole life. It doesn't require words; it just is. Love for self, love for family, love for close friends, love for people I meet, love I share through hands-on or through directing is a never-ending stream. TRT® provides a connection to the many levels of myself and the many levels of others and God, universal energy. I even feel one with people who have physically died. I know they are a part of the whole and part of me."

Insights on Death and Dying

Being at the bedside of a dying person provides the opportunity for reflection about personal beliefs and views around death and dying. It also can trigger feelings and emotions from experiences that are still present. "My TRT® training helped me deal with my past experiences and feelings toward death," shares Don Bates. "I was eight years old when one of my brothers died suddenly of a brain tumour. I cannot remember the funeral. All I can remember is being in a car at the cemetery. I wanted to cry, but I did not. My family were very private and we did not show our emotions. I realized how much I have grown and the process continues. The Radiance Technique® has opened a whole new world.

"Thinking of dying and preparing for dying is not something that I dwell on. However, being in the moment, touching another person, and even smelling a flower has taken on a deeper meaning for me. TRT® has given me something special, a connection to my inner self."

By practicing TRT® on an ongoing basis, shifts in perception and how we view things can change. It does not happen overnight. Sherry Brunelle shares, "Recently, my hands-on sessions helped me to focus on my dad's dying in peace as opposed to his death. This was very healing for me."

Hands-on meditations also supported John Bondy: "Through TRT®, I have come to terms with my own death, and I feel the continuum between life and death is more of a flow to a different dimension," he reveals. "It has helped me come to terms with my parents' death. I actually feel close to my parents again since their death."

For Rita Lepp, a volunteer since 1994, a profound realization took place: "Since studying and practicing TRT®, my perception of life has broadened in many areas. I have a more positive and joyful outlook of daily life and a less morbid perception of death. Death is not an end but a transition."

June Middleton has experienced healing around the death of her husband. "In the summer of '92, Bill and I shared two weeks vacation with my kid brother and his wife. Bill commented it was the best vacation he had ever had. We did notice that he had a cough all winter and into the summer. After a visit to the doctor and many tests, he received the diagnosis of lung cancer. We were hoping to have a miracle. It wasn't to be. Bill died at home on February 27, 1993. How could this be? He was only 67. Yet I knew it was for the best; down the road, the pain would have been unbearable for him.

"The experience left a huge hole in me; half of me was lost, feeling grief. The other half of me was filled with anger, of what if? Why? So many feelings. We would have been married 44 years that summer. Now the 17th anniversary of his death is approaching.

"Our TRT® training on death and dying triggered a lot of emotions within me. It was like the flood gates opened. It was very healing. I still miss Bill. Moreover, I have grown. I have grown more with TRT®.

"I had been doing TRT® sessions regularly since our classes began. Sometimes we do not realize we are tense or stressed. I did not think I was. What source of stress did I have? However, here I was feeling more relaxed... Ah! The calm within me was my greatest discovery and gift.

"I experienced tingling in my fingers, which progressed into fingers and thumbs, then all of my hand, the back of hands, my lips. Then my hands on my body felt weightless; even the blankets were weightless. My toes tingled, and the bottom of my feet — amazing. 'Wow, I am just one big tingle,' I thought.

"After reading *The Radiance Technique® and AIDS*, I assumed the proper word for this tingling was vibrations. From my own daily hands-on sessions, I observed that while reading I had complete concentration. No monkey mind. Wow! It was amazing to read how TRT®is giving so many comfort and love."

Expanding Caring Qualities

There is no question that volunteers feel better from having a method to release tension, restore energy and provide deep rest. It enables them to respond to the stress in their lives in a more balanced, healthy way. In addition to physical and mental benefits, consistent and daily practice of TRT® improves their quality of life and supports their transformation to become a more peaceful and kind human being. It does this by connecting directly to a higher order of Light energy and aligning this energy from within. Experiencing inner peace is the basis for all higher levels of consciousness. Volunteers are able to carry that quality of deep *Radiant Peace*sm in everything that they do. With TRT®, volunteers are able to generate the deeper qualities of caring, compassion and unconditional love.

> *It has been said for centuries that love is the best healer and wholer. Love is a quality of the life-force, and TRT® accesses Universal Love, Radiant energy. Love is not something you create. It is your True nature. For centuries, those who have been wise and awake have reminded us that we are Love and Light in this world. TRT® brings a gift of Light-energy that aligns you with your inner, natural integrity.*[2]

Compassion in Action

Volunteers step forward to enhance people's quality of life without regard for recognition, reward or financial gain. Compassion in action is the genuine act of giving rather than getting. We can never put a value on what volunteers do.

Their benevolence is priceless. If you ask any volunteer, you will hear them say over and over again how they feel they receive much more from volunteering than they feel they give.

"I came to Hospice because I wanted to give back something to the community," says Don Bates. "I've tried other things but Hospice was the thing that touched me the most. On our first day of TRT® classes, our teacher asked us to write the answer to the following question in our journal, 'Why are you here?' I wrote that I was open to receiving more connection to my inner self. I wanted to be the most I could be on a spiritual level. I have always enjoyed the poem *Footprints in the Sand.* Our journey through life is not always easy, but I know in my life God has carried me many times, and if it were not for Him and others, I would not be who I am today. I wanted a way I could give back to others and I feel TRT® is my answer.

"The Radiance Technique® has and continues to amaze me. When I share TRT®, the peace I feel provides the spirit of tranquility, which is both comforting and renewing. It is uplifting to see others after a session relax and sometimes have a glow about them. I see the relaxation and the calmness in a person's face when I am doing a session. I am giving back something special. I find that I, too, receive rest and relaxation. It is a win-win situation. How can you beat that?"

For Rita, TRT® became a way to expand her caregiving capacity: "Before studying TRT®, I knew that I was a good volunteer who supported and listened to patients while visiting them in the hospital or home. However, I felt there was little I could do to change or help their current situation or condition. Now, I have added another dimension to my service by communicating at a deeper level.

"I remember a special patient, Mr. Myers, who was diagnosed with colon cancer at the age of 50. I sensed I needed to visit him every other day as he was failing quickly and felt that the end of his physical existence was near. During our last session, Mr. Myers said, 'It was so beautiful.' He was speaking of 'somewhere else.' I did not comment and completed our session together with my hands on his heart. This was a very moving experience for me. He died a few hours later after going into a coma.

"Experiences like this convince me that another dimension of communication is taking place. This gives me the assurance and confidence to continue practicing TRT® without expecting to see certain results. I truly believe that TRT® addresses the greatest needs of each individual.

"At the age of 70, I now have a deeper understanding of caregiving, and my capacity for being with patients has expanded. During hands-on or directing, there is an unspoken communication and connection. Even though some may not be aware of it, I know that TRT® is helping them. I support them silently and joyously on their journey."

For Pat Bachand, The Radiance Technique® is a sacred energy and a gift to be shared. Her experiences inspired her to become an Authorized Instructor of The First Degree Official Program of TRT®, Authentic Reiki®. She volunteers at the Wellness Centre and describes what TRT® has done for her life.

"Part of my daily prayer is 'Lord, I ask that I be your shepherd and gather your flock.' TRT® answered this prayer. Having TRT® in my life has heightened my awareness, with gratitude, love and compassion.

"The Radiance Technique® has changed my life beyond all my expectations. It allows me to be present with each unfolding moment of continual rebirth. It allows me to connect with my authentic self, the discovery and reconnecting of my original blueprint.

"I most often use Head Positions for headaches and stress and Front Position #1 for sadness, grief and difficult times. When I need strength and direction to be all that I can be, I place my hands on Front Position #2 and use Cosmic Symbols and Attunements.

"On my half hour drive to the Centre I pray and then direct Radiant energy to each client and to anyone who comes into the room. I give thanks for this day, this time in my life and the gift of TRT®.

"The awakening and connecting with my intuition and visualizations has been a precious gift that has often allowed me to share in a greater healing with clients. No two sessions are ever the same. Our needs and our energy are always different. Each session is a tremendous gift as well as an experience.

"To see and share in the awakening and spiritual growth of each client from the first session to the fourth session is a magnificent, sacred gift. A woman in her 50s once told me, 'I think I have been asleep all my life. I feel lighter, awake, connected — even the colours around me are so much brighter.'

"Radiant energy is a rebirth into the next moment, a continuum, an interconnectedness to all that is. One of love, honour and sacredness. The gifts I receive each day continue to reach beyond all my expectations."

Simply Being With

Long time volunteer, Pat Barton recalls, "I had two remarkable experiences of really 'being with' someone. During a Radiant Touch® session, my hands felt as if they entered the patient's body. It is hard to explain; it felt as if my hands just sank beneath the skin, and I could feel the current of life energy flowing through them. This was an amazing experience for me.

"Without exception, every person I have shared TRT® with felt better. I remember two clients in particular who were in extreme pain, and the sessions helped tremendously. Two months later, one client is still experiencing unusual relief in her neck. The other had a crushed heel from an accident 25 years ago and has had two surgeries but is always in pain. He claimed he could feel his ankle give two 'clicks' while my hands were on Head Position #1, and the pain disappeared. He still felt no pain six days later, something he had never experienced before. I do not try to explain it; I just let it be. Radiant Touch® is a pleasure to do for others; it is relaxing for the giver as well as the receiver."

June echoes Pats appreciation, and she continues to be in awe about her experiences: "The reactions and comments I've received giving sessions of TRT® to other people leave me in awe," she says. "Some feedback is given from family, acquaintances and others who are strangers. I am amazed at their complete relaxation, their stillness, and their trust. Their gentle snoring makes me smile. I feel privileged and honoured at their trust and they say, 'An hour already? I feel so relaxed, the headache I had is gone. Did I sleep? I feel rested, I'd like some more, my arthritis wasn't as bad the next morning, Oh, I went back to my childhood and visited my family...', and the comments continue.

"I feel so blessed that I can share The Radiance Technique®, to share a bit of comfort and love, some peace, calm and relaxation — to help others experience the quiet within them. I have personally felt all of these changes since practicing hands-on every day. I am happier and I continue to grow."

Expanding Inner Service

Volunteers with The Second Degree level of training or higher, utilize methods to expand their service and support to patients beyond their bedside. These techniques enable volunteers to "direct" energy to others beyond time and space. A few examples include when the volunteer cannot physically be there, like during surgery, before, and after their volunteer visits. This inner contribution is an ongoing service many volunteers daily employ.

Rita shares about her expansion of inner contributions to others while using TRT®: "The Second Degree has taken me a step further. I am not limited to time and space. I can connect with a person anytime, anywhere; there are no limits. I have my ever-expanding radiant list of people, which includes new patients and family members and friends that I include in my daily directing. If someone dies, I record the date of their transition, and they remain on my list, continuing to receive energy support."

For John Brownlie, continuing in his studies of TRT® opened up a whole new way of being: "My sessions both with clients and for myself, took a quantum leap after completing The Second Degree. I remember the instructor talking about the value of 'being with'. At the time, I did not really know what this meant, although I convinced myself that I had a general idea. It was several weeks later that I truly experienced the feeling of 'being with' someone.

"I was assigned to a patient in the hospital who had carcinoma of the throat. He was bleeding internally, the source of which could not be located. His wife informed me that he had been taken off all support and was being medicated regularly to control any pain. His daughter had experienced TRT® and felt that it would calm and relax her father.

"I began the 12 positions. While at Front Position #3, I became subtly aware of a sense of calm. The two of us together were in the peace and tranquillity of another place of peace. A little voice inside me was saying, 'OK, let's move on to the next position,' but I had no desire to move. I stayed right there. It felt so right to continue this feeling of immense calm, I just went with the feeling. Eventually, I did move to Front Position #4, and this wonderful feeling of calm stillness was even stronger. The feeling was not requesting anything, not achieving anything, just being. Again, I stayed right there.

"I now realize that this was my first experience of 'being with' someone. It was like being somewhere and being nowhere at the same time. My hands were there; my attention was there and then a subtle shift occurs from listening with my hands, to listening with my whole being. This is a shift from being there with my hands to being there with my whole self.

"The physical world dissolves; no room, no bed, and no patient, no me. I am only aware of the energy, a melting together of energies, not his, not mine, just one energy that floats in space, not attached to anything or anyone.

"It is in this profound stillness, this profound oneness that I really connect on an inner plane with another person. Nothing is said, nothing is done — just being there, listening with my whole self. It is a very rewarding experience.

"I am learning now that 'being with' can extend to anything I desire to experience in radiant stillness: a tree, a whole forest, a situation. Before me lies a whole world to explore and I can't wait to begin."

The Radiance Technique is more than a technique for volunteers and, for Melanie Johnson, TRT® has become a part of her life, her home, her work and her service to others. She sums up her feelings about TRT® as "coming home."

"The Second Degree of TRT® was like an awakening for me. It opened up countless avenues for healing and loving," she relates. "These avenues extend beyond time and space into all facets of life — past, present and future. I wanted to take The Second Degree Official Program of The Radiance Technique®, Authentic Reiki® to enhance my work with Hospice patients and to light up my own life, and indeed, it did. I now have the ability to direct Radiant energy to any part of my life. It enhances and supports my working relationships with my coworkers and community partners. It enhances my relationships with my family, friends and Hospice patients. In fact, because TRT® is not limited by time or space, I am able to direct TRT® backward in time to support past conflicts, illnesses, difficult situations and past hurts. There is no relationship, experience or situation that cannot be transformed.

"I use this ability to direct TRT® to Hospice patients prior to my visit with them. In this way, our meeting is already radiantly supported by the time I arrive.

"I have received the benefits of directing by others. My Radiant Touch® team at Hospice supported me prior to and during a very serious surgery. Those who had The Second Degree and beyond directed TRT® to me in the hospital and during my recovery. They were not able to be physically present because the hospital was four hundred kilometres away. The pace of my recovery has been exceptional, and this amazes those who know me. I have had three previous abdominal surgeries and, this being the fourth, was by far the most invasive and complicated of the bunch. With the inner support of TRT®, I have also had less pain.

"I have continued my expansion and I am now an Authorized Instructor of The First Degree Official Program of The Radiance Technique®, Authentic Reiki®. This expansion has been like emerging from a cocoon into trans-formation.

"I have heard it said that when you travel with someone, you truly get to know them. I am truly getting to know myself on this radiantly supported journey. I am seeing and experi-encing the joy in life's challenges rather than blocking the joy with fear. The challenges of life may be harder and more com-plex, but through The Radiance Technique®, I am living it easier.

"I am amazed with the expansion through each degree, how each level offers more depth, more gifts. This expansion has enhanced the sessions with my Hospice patients. I am able to move through difficult situations with greater ease. People are responding to me more positively. I bring a more centred and attentive persona to each session.

"Seven years ago, I was dying. I had one foot in the grave. Today, together with The Radiance Technique® and medical science, my health is restored. I feel younger than I did a decade ago. There are limitless possibilities for ways to direct and expand with TRT® to benefit everyone and everything. TRT® has become a part of my life; I use it automatically and continuously. I do not know how I got up out of bed without it! I am turning into the light — around and around into the light." Radiant Touch® volunteers are spiritual comforters providing a vital contribution to our community's well-being. Alongside the Hospice health care team, they are valuable members who make a difference. Many of these volunteers share additional experiences face to face in the companion DVD. Hospice palliative care combines active and compassionate therapies intended to comfort and support individuals and their friends and families who are living with or dying from a life-threatening illness.

[1] Barbara Ray, Ph.D. with Shoshana Shay, comp., 'This Moment in Time,' The Awakening Journey® Day by Day, Selections from the Teachings of Dr. Barbara Ray. (St. Petersburg, FL: Radiance Associates, 2002) October 12.

[2] Barbara Ray, Ph.D., The 'Reiki' Factor in The Radiance Technique® Expanded Edition, (St. Petersburg, FL: Radiance Associates, 1992), p. 114.

PART 2

Be a light unto yourself.

~ Buddha

The Healing Journey

My journey with cancer is...
an opportunity for me to experience
the <u>Real</u> meaning of wellness and of <u>life</u>!
And The Radiance Technique®
has been the key which opens the doors
of experience and understanding. ...[1]

~ Katherine Lenel,
"The Radiance Technique® and Cancer"
Authorized Instructor of The Radiance Technique®

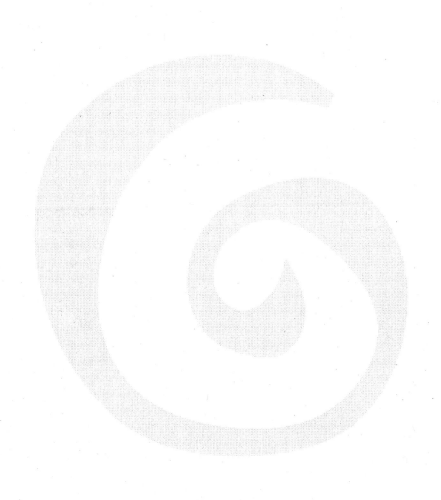

-3-

No matter what is happening physically, the opportunity to experience well-being is possible with the nurturing support of The Radiance Technique®. The energy capacities of TRT® provide many stress relieving benefits. Whether upon first hearing news of diagnosis to experiencing the challenges that come, people experience this transcendental energy and have used it in various ways to cope, to heal and experience a higher quality of life. This chapter highlights sharings from Windsor and also includes experiences from practitioners in England, Greece and the United States.

TRT® and Lymphoma: Personal Journeys to Wellness

An Interview with Katherine Lenel

Katherine Lenel is an Authorized Instructor of TRT® and the author of *The Radiance Technique® and Cancer*. In this book, she takes us through her courageous journey with cancer from diagnosis through the completion of her chemo and explains how she used TRT® as a support system at all stages of the process. Her account also includes sharings from other cancer survivors and from people's experiences of supporting Katherine through TRT® hands-on and regularly directed Radiant energy. She is thriving 15 years after her diagnosis of non-Hodgkin's lymphoma. Katherine is now leading a full and active life. In her book she writes, *"My journey with cancer is... an opportunity for me to experience the Real meaning of wellness and of life! And The Radiance Technique® has been the key which opens the doors of experience and understanding.*"[2] Katherine has now studied to The Seventh Degree and shared further insights in the following interview.

Christine Maria Gross: How do you use TRT® as part of your wellness program or as a method of prevention?

Katherine Lenel: I use TRT® hands-on for about an hour nearly every morning and until I fall asleep at night. I also direct energy as I learned in a TRT® seminar, using Cosmic Symbols, every morning and evening. I find it helps to energize me in the morning, settle me down in the evening, and connect with and care for my world before and after my daily life activities in the outer world. I usually direct energy to Radiant Peace[sm] on the planet at noon each day.

Q: Do you feel the use of TRT® has had any impact on your immune system? Or that TRT® has extended your length of life?

Katherine: Yes, I do. At this time, I am 15 years in remission, and I experience my level of health and well-being as strong and perhaps more stable than before my illness. I have learned how to nurture myself so that while I understand that a year of chemotherapy has likely compromised my immune system, I am not especially aware of being unable to do what I choose to do, and I do not seem more than normally susceptible to the illnesses of others around me.

Q: How did TRT® assist you with treatments like chemotherapy and drug therapies?

Katherine: I experienced chemotherapy as very draining to my energy. I used TRT® while lying down on a cot in my office between the classes I taught at the University of Miami. I usually had about a half an hour and I used the time for Head Positions #1, #2, #3, #4 and Front Positions #1 and #3. I regained enough energy to be ready to teach my next class. I also used hands-on with the oral chemotherapy drugs that I took for one out of every three weeks for a year. I held the pills in my hands for five to ten minutes before swallowing them.

Q: Has TRT® changed your quality of life? Is your life different from pre-TRT®?

Katherine: The gradual calming and settling down, the increasing ability to take things as they come, to choose to do what seems good to me, to recognize my connection with people and the world in which I live, to sense when it is "time" to act, or to rest — all of these seem connected to my use of TRT®.

The quality of my life since TRT® has risen in stability, flexibility, humour, joy and a well-being that is not tied to my physical health though that has also been mostly very good. What impresses me the most is that these changes seem to have occurred not because I told my self to change, not because I tried to "get better", but as if unfolding naturally, with less and less strain and effort, with more and more acceptance and ease, in relation to my everyday use of The Radiance Technique®.

Q: Has TRT® expanded your understanding and experience of energy within you and around you?

Katherine: Yes. I feel things in a way I never noticed before. I can identify my feelings and sense of things inside me and also coming from other people and events. I can allow these feelings and "senses of things" to grow in me until I know how to respond. I could never do that in my childhood or young adulthood. I can also tell the difference between thoughts, emotions and sensations. I am aware of an inner sense of silence, fullness, and Radiant Peace[sm], more than I have been at any other time of life. My sense of the wonder of life is greater than ever before.

Q: Has TRT® helped you handle emotions?

Katherine: The Radiance Technique® has helped me to begin to observe my emotions, painful and joyous, without judging them and so to have the "space" to respond to them in a way that allows me to make choices in behaviour that serve myself, without having to act upon it immediately. This is making a tremendous difference in my enjoyment of my life and, I think, in my effectiveness in everything I do. TRT® Hands-on and the technique for directing energy in addition to the use of the hands, co-create that "space" for me to observe and "be with" what I am feeling in a state or atmosphere of acceptance and interest, without panic or anger.

Q: Has TRT® given you any insights into the healing/wholing process?

Katherine: The most important thing I believe I have learned about the healing/wholing process through TRT® is that I can be really "well" even when I am feeling sick. Using TRT® has come a long way to release me from the fear I always felt when ill — fear that I couldn't do what I wanted to do, that I would never recover, that now illness was all that was real. It helped me develop a broader view, again, without asking me to believe in any written or spoken idea about anything, that allowed me to see what I was experiencing more clearly and without the projections and interpretations I grew up attaching to illness and disability.

Q: Does the Radiant energy of TRT® help you feel more nurturing, accepting and compassionate towards yourself and others?

Katherine: Yes, most definitely. In my perception, the gentleness and warmth of this Radiant energy just naturally fosters or generates the experience of acceptance, nurturing and compassion so that the more I use TRT®, the more those qualities or energies become a natural part of my living experience. Not because I try to accept or nurture others, or myself, but because that just becomes the natural thing to do.

Q: How do you view the cycles of life of birthing and dying?

Katherine: Since my experience with cancer and my use of TRT® in conjunction with my illness, I am more aware that my life on this earth is an opportunity to awaken, that every action or non-action is a choice that creates more or less Light and Aliveness for me and for everyone. I don't believe I ever had the least sense of this truth before TRT®. I still work with what that really means moment to moment, but it has made my view of life and death much richer and fuller than I ever knew in the past."

In the following, Dr. Barbara Ray offers insights on the qualities of being well, no matter what is going on physically:

Well — Refers to your state of being and the harmony and balance of your physical, emotional and mental planes and the awareness you have of the interrelationship of the inner and outer planes of your Being. "Being well" is a quality of the energy of wholeness — not a partial aspect of yourself such as not being sick on the physical plane. Your "wellness" includes the whole of you and includes such aspects as the physical body, your feelings, your mental capacities, your zest for living, your enthusiasm for learning or exploring the movement into the unknown, your capacity for self-awareness, your behaviors — all that you manifest on the outer planes of your existence which deeply interconnects to your awareness of your inner planes and your capacity for higher consciousness and spiritual awakening. ...[3]

TRT and Inner Strength

In this sharing, Delores Paolatto describes how TRT® helped her through her lymphoma diagnosis, recurrence and end-of-life. "I have made TRT® a part of my daily activities. Each morning after I complete my Radiant Touch® session, I no longer feel any stiffness and chest pains usually felt when I was awake. As I do TRT® each morning, I can feel the warmth generating from my hands and body in different positions, and I can experience my blood flow increasing and revitalizing that particular area.

"This technique has taught me to help myself in gaining more confidence. TRT® has decreased my level of anxiety and fear involving minor situations that most people take for granted. For example, I am not driving a car on my own and am taking the initiative to do things without family members being there supporting me like going grocery shopping, attending social events and activities. Emotionally, I have grown more tolerant and assured. TRT® is providing me with an inner strength and calmness. It helps me to have a more positive outlook on life."

Empowerment

Barbara Mahoney had two close friends who were diagnosed with breast cancer at the same time she received the news of her diagnosis. It was very difficult for her as she witnessed them getting weaker and eventually dying. I remember her saying, "Why am I still alive?" Over a period of time, her TRT® sessions supported her to have less fear of the future and a heightened ability to recognize that she had resources to heal and empower herself.

"My introduction to The Radiance Technique® came about as a result of a referral to Hospice," says Barbara. "The referral was preceded by a diagnosis of non-Hodgkin's lymphoma in the orbit area of my right eye. Consequently, my experience with TRT® of three sets of four sessions given at weekly intervals at the Wellness Centre.

"The first set began the week that I completed a series of radiation treatments — from today's perspective I realize that I was very much in battle mode — fighting a war against cancer. Fear and confusion were dominant, but I did not have the time or the energy to work with either. Survival required that I simply get through each day as well as possible. Getting through the day usually meant going to work, coming home, resting for a short time, eating and then retiring for the night. Fatigue was ever present and my prayers routinely asked for the strength to complete each day's tasks and to find the time needed to rest and heal. The Radiant Touch® sessions during this initial healing time were a source of comfort, a safe place in which to simply be. The sessions were also a time when I could seem to go to a deeper place to rest and find a calm quiet oasis. The fatigue was ever-present and so overwhelming that even resting did not provide relief. There were times when the fatigue itself seemed to block sleep. In the midst of this struggle (needing rest desperately, but often not able to even sleep), the Radiant Touch® sessions were most welcomed, a refuge from the struggle. Many times, I simply wanted to remain on the table at the completion of the session. At times, I felt as if the table and I were one. I seemed to sink into the table and there was no perception of separation between the table and myself.

"The second set of sessions took place three months later. While the fatigue had lessened, it was still sufficiently present to be bothersome. As well, my employment had ended, and I was experiencing a deep sense of loss. At times, I felt as though my world was disintegrating and I was powerless to stop the process. The future was becoming too uncertain to contemplate. During this period, the sessions provided a peaceful respite. The appointments provided structure when it seemed as if all the structure in my life had simply dissolved. The simple act of entering the radiant space was soothing. The peaceful energy in the room seemed to penetrate my very being and took me to a quieter inner state. Before each session, Christine provided time to talk, and I looked forward to these times as I was attempting to gain some sense of my life in the midst of very serious changes. Again, the sense of deep relaxation and of seeming to sink into the table added to my healing process. For a short time at least, my tears and worries were set aside, and I could go within, secure in the presence of the Radiant energy.

"Approximately three weeks later, I began my last set of sessions. These sessions were instructional in nature and required my participation at a more viable level. Personally, this was a time when the fatigue had become more of a minor problem and my energy was being felt more consistently. The nature of the sessions and my own healing process were well-matched. As well, I knew that I wanted the effects of TRT® to continue in my life, and so I welcomed the offer to learn The First Degree Official Program of The Radiance Technique®, Authentic Reiki®.

"I was, and still am, in an up-and-down period in my life wondering what the future will hold, taking sometimes tentative steps to build a secure future while fighting the old demons of fear, passivity and low self-esteem. My whole being had been shaken to its core. I knew that I had to go within to find the strength to work through this period of transition. The First Degree has given me a source of empowering energy that can be activated when needed.

• "The initial appointments were about surviving and simply getting through a most difficult time. The later sessions brought a sense of peace and calm. They seemed to fill me with a warm glow; they nourished my soul. While it was with regret that I left the last session, I knew that I was not leaving TRT®. Rather, I knew that its energy and positive effects would continue to enhance my life.

"My experience with TRT® has been a time of healing, change and growth. So much had happened and so much had left my life in a short period of time. I felt rootless and lost. I was too tired to practice my usual methods of healing: meditating, walking, writing, sharing with dear friends. TRT® filled the void. There were times in the initial sessions when I wondered if I would have the energy to attend a session. I was always happy that I managed to do so.

"I currently use TRT® in the morning at least four to five times a week and occasionally at night. I find that using it gives me a deepening sense of peace. It brings a calm that helps me adapt to the changes that are still ongoing in my life. The practice of TRT® assists in the cleansing of negative thoughts and feelings and contributes to the developing sense that I can go on to effect the necessary changes in my life. It has further proven the old adage that when one door closes, another door opens. I am grateful that the doorway to The Radiance Technique® opened and I intend to continue deepening my experience with it."

TRT® and Breast Cancer: Five Stories of Courage

A cancer diagnosis may be initially frightening and overwhelming. For women, probably the most challenging diagnosis is that of breast cancer. Breast cancer affects many women and is prevalent in high numbers in our society. Statistics for breast cancer in Canadian women (estimated) for 2007 are 22,300 new diagnoses.[4] Breasts are symbolic of the feminine, and having a breast surgically removed is not only physically traumatic but psychologically and emotionally traumatic as well. Dealing with the after-effects of body image and sexuality can cause anxiety and depression. The following five women share their real experiences.

Susan Hess is a breast cancer activist, advocate and survivor. At the time of her diagnosis, she was a widowed mother of five. Today, Susan is an inspiration to many. Her journey brought her to become President of Willow Breast Cancer Support and Resources Services. Willow is an organization that provides survivor-to-survivor emotional support and information about breast cancer to anyone in Canada. Susan has made amazing contributions in supporting and bringing awareness to our community and beyond. "My Radiant Touch® sessions took me to a place of deep peace and calm," she explains, "so that my body was in the most relaxed state to be able to accept the chemotherapy needed to fight the disease. It also allowed me a one-hour holiday that lasted many hours — freeing my mind of the worry that cluttered its corridors.

"I later studied The First Degree Official Program of The Radiance Technique®, Authentic Reiki® and learned to apply this for myself. Being able to provide TRT® to others faced with breast cancer surgery has been a gift. I have seen women almost paralyzed with fear, strung tighter than a drum, fall into a deep sleep. In fact, one husband called me to say, 'I do not know what you did. Thank you because last night (which happened to be the night before her double mastectomy), she slept like a baby. It was the first time in five days.' What greater gift can you give and can you receive than that!"

For eight years, Lyn Turner lived as a breast cancer survivor. She was Susan's friend and came full circle as an active participant in her own health and in her community. Lyn was a member of the dragon boat team called *A Breast or Knot,* showed her smiling face in March of the 2005 calendar *Beauty Beyond Breast Cancer* and had supported women in finding a life outside of cancer by also volunteering as a facilitator in local breast cancer groups. She studied to The Second Degree and, as a Radiant Touch® volunteer, Lyn offered her personal experience and support to many patients. She was an inspiration to all.

"My very first contact with TRT® was a week after my diagnosis when I contacted my neighbour Susan who had undergone a similar experience some years earlier," she shares. "I was, needless to say, very distraught, my mind swirling with information about breast cancer. My mother had died of breast cancer 25 years ago. Susan offered me this relaxation session and I accepted. I seemed to be soothed and felt quite drawn to this energy; the session seemed to strike a chord in my being.

"After my mastectomy surgery, I came to Hospice to attend supportive programs and one of the programs offered to me was Radiant Touch®. I am thankful for the sessions I had while undergoing chemotherapy and radiation. These sessions gave me the energy to endure treatment and the understanding to help heal myself.

"Training in TRT® was offered through Hospice and both my husband and I participated. Studying it together gave us an opportunity to be with each other, to experience a sharing and healing time. It was something pleasant to share during my treatment phase, and I supported my husband in his anxiety and mourning of his mother's death at the time of my diagnosis.

"Using TRT® at home daily helped me emotionally and physically. People would tell me that I was doing very well because I didn't experience nausea. I attribute it to this self-help technique, which I gave myself at least twice if not three times a day. I was quite upbeat and strong.

"TRT® still helps me personally. I have been using it for seven years now and it continues to help me remain balanced. It has been a real grounding to keep me going and has enabled me to stay well. For example, when I have a hectic day, a 20-minute hands-on session will literally pick me up and help me continue the day.

"Lymphedema is a side effect from surgery and I find sessions help reduce the swelling noticeably. I have found the following positions to be supportive for lymphatic drainage: Head Position #4, and Front Positions #1 and #4.

"I often find my hand on my heart position while reading or watching television and while in the car. In the quiet of the house or on a walk, I have been paying attention to my feelings and contemplating where I want to go and what is important to me. I also share with friends, and once they have received a session of TRT®, they have requested another spot to be set aside for them.

"As a Hospice volunteer, I completed additional training to provide sessions to Hospice clients. It has enabled me to touch and support people on all levels — body, mind, emotion and spirit. It has enabled me to touch people, in that I can sense when they need help and there is a deeper awareness, a sort of 'tuning in' that I have never noticed before. I feel honoured to help others in their journey to a place of relaxation and peace using The Radiance Technique® as it has and continues to support me."

Support to Trust My Body

At the age of 53, KeriAnn Mahoney, R.N., M.A., was diagnosed with breast cancer. After her lumpectomy, she was referred to Hospice for support. When I first met KeriAnn, she told me that she had lost faith in her body. She also suffered from chronic fatigue syndrome, and had been involved in a few car accidents in the past ten years, one of which resulted in her left side being paralyzed. She recovered but continued to be plagued by pain.

"First of all, I want to point out that I come from a traditional medical background, along with years of previous training and experience with other energy therapies such as Therapeutic Touch™, healing touch, polarity and bioenergetics, to name a few. What I like about TRT® is how gentle it is and how easy it is to use for self-healing. During my journey with cancer, TRT® empowered me to feel a part of my oncology team. Now I use it to support myself during other health challenges.

"Working with Christine early in my journey with cancer helped me realize that I had to make a choice: Would I choose life-enhancing activities which brought me joy, peace and tranquillity; or would I continue to choose stressful activities which I believe would feed cancer, inevitably resulting in my death? I knew I had a choice, and even today, I continue to grapple with which choices are life-enhancing. For me, working with TRT® facilitates conscious awareness of my options. It also helps me negotiate between social expectations and my physical needs. It continues to support and facilitate my personal process through life challenges.

"I treasured the opportunity of having TRT® to help me regain a little composure, balance and focus during such a stressful time in my life. I firmly believe that this subtle energy work empowers patients to make choices that are more appropriate and to work more easily with medical decisions. Simply, it makes a person's journey with cancer much smoother.

"TRT® enabled me to cry a lot, feel my fears and release emotional prejudices about cancer. It helps me work with my emotions to facilitate them, release them, integrate them and restore balance and harmony. Currently, I am caught in a modern belief system about disease that creates guilt and shame about illness for me. Working with TRT® helps me view disease as a process rather than the direct result of negative thoughts and childhood experiences. Rather than perceiving it as punishment, I am beginning to allow myself the 'gift' of disease as a natural process, simply a component of our human journey. I continue to find this a very difficult issue to transform and integrate. TRT® helps me to move through any emotional process — anger, fear, grief, anxiety — to restore inner harmony.

"I used TRT® on myself during the period of radiation treatments: while waiting for actual treatments, while driving myself to treatments and appointments and while waiting test results. It relieves my stress and supports me through challenges. Today, I continue to use it during magnetic drum therapy sessions through my chiropractor.

"I can use TRT® no matter how much weakness, fatigue and pain I am facing. It makes me more aware of my body and affords me a tool to work with my own subtle energies. It has become an integral component of my personal wellness program. Its use relaxes and empowers me to focus on healing when I feel unwell.

"Because I tend to carry stress in my lung and diaphragm areas, I usually draw on TRT®'s Front Positions. As well, I utilize Head Positions to ameliorate mental confusion and restore relaxation. Positions I use for chronic pain depend upon location and severity. For example, when jaw pain is serious, I use Head Positions #2, #3 and #4. For back and shoulder pain, I employ Front #3 and #4 and the back positions.

"The TRT®'s reservoir concept helps me see the human body in a different way. It makes me aware of the need to take responsibility for my body's need for rest and relaxation. The hands-on positions give me a specific and gentle process to follow which enables that rest to happen on a very deep level.

"In a nutshell, TRT® gives me hope. Although I have a number of skills to help me journey with cancer, the primary difference is that I can use TRT® independently or in combination with others with ease. Has TRT® helped me find meaning in my life? The Radiance Technique® has helped me *have* a life. I'm still integrating the fact of having survived cancer. Recently, I completed training in The Second Degree. I like how it supports life in the here and now and helps me accept and trust in my body's messages to me."

Support During Reconstruction Surgery

Carol embraced TRT® as a constant support for her journey. After all of her treatments and surgery were completed, she became a volunteer at Grace Hospital in the neonatal unit. Her job? Touching, holding and feeding babies with her radiant hands.

"I first experienced The Radiance Technique® late in 1994. I had gone through many surgeries, radiation and chemotherapy to treat breast cancer. I was preparing for a six-hour reconstruction surgery scheduled for Fall of '95. I wanted the reconstruction so my body would be whole again. I was aware of the toll the treatments were taking on me and wanted to be as strong and peaceful as I could be for the future surgery. I felt my soul, along with my body, had been scarred also. I needed to repair that, to become complete spiritually and emotionally.

"The following is a quote from my journal for December 1, 1994. It best describes one of my most memorable experiences with The Radiance Technique®. *When Christine put her hands on my temples, I felt my mother's touch as sure as if she was in the room, as sure as if it were her hands on my head. I felt her touch. I remember her hands, soft, loving, gentle. I remember her touch. I remember her now. I can feel her touch. I can see her hands. I can remember the feel of her hands. I remember her love. For so long I had forgotten and now I remember.*

"Other memorable sessions included me looking down from the ceiling and watching Christine share Radiant Touch® with me. This gave me the opportunity to view myself from a more enlightened place. Other times, I felt my whole body being energized. My skin felt hot and dry, and Christine's hands were cool and calming like touching cool shaded grass in the middle of a hot summer's day.

"I always felt that something had changed within me after each session, although I cannot put words to it. I cannot describe the change. It was very deep within my core. I always felt peaceful, relaxed and happy after my sessions. It had been a few years since I had had any peace at all.

"I took The First Degree Official Program of The Radiance Technique®, Authentic Reiki® later that year. I was then able to do TRT® on myself. This was very useful in preparing for my upcoming surgery. Along with my ongoing sessions with Christine, I would do sessions on myself daily, with extra time on the surgical areas.

"I feel that The Radiance Technique® prepared me for what has so far been my last surgery. It prepared my body and soul. My surgery was uncomplicated. I had no pain. The hospital staff remarked that I required only minimal pain medication. I was up and walking the hallways the very next day. That is remarkable in itself considering the incisions that I had.

"In the hospital and at home afterwards, I slept mostly all day and night. I would put my hands in one of the front positions while sleeping, and I would wake many hours later in the same position. I was healing rapidly. The sleep felt calming, healing and spiritual. I know TRT® had caused that. Following previous surgeries, my recuperation period was unpleasant. The sleep I did get was not restful. I was jumpy, anxious and unhappy.

"I believe The Radiance Technique® has healed me physically and spiritually. It has allowed me to feel connected to a higher energy, to the universe. It has shaped my beliefs so that I am no longer connected to the outcome of a situation. It has allowed me to experience the belief that I can be in a higher place regardless of what is happening around me. It has allowed me to nurture my physical body. It has allowed me to expand my soul. I am grateful for this experience. I am grateful for being whole again.

"I feel this peace and calmness have an effect on my body. I believe these feelings affect my immune system in a positive way. My sleep is restorative; my energy is not wasted in nega-tivity. Sometimes my skin glows with radiance. Other people notice this glowing. Some ask if I am hot. I am hot, not physi-cally, but glowing with Radiant energy that is flowing from the universe through my heart and soul. A true blessing.

"Mostly, I am grateful that The Radiance Technique® has allowed a spiritual connection for me to my mother and also with God. Many times since my first experience, I have again felt her touch. I have felt the presence of God, my belief of God, a universal energy, one to which we are all connected to, a peaceful light, one that shines always. I am grateful that my eyes were opened by The Radiance Technique® so that I am able to see this light, to experience this peace."

TRT® provides deep rest and relaxation for the recovery process. On the subject of recovery, Dr. Barbara Ray offers the following:

> *Recovering Process — Refers to returning to a balanced range of energy; to stabilize in a more whole, balanced condition. You can be recovering — i.e., regaining stability — on any of your outer planes of the physical-emotional-mental dynamic in a healing/wholing process. The Radiance Technique® is an invaluable tool for transformation, for returning balancing, restoring wholing energy and for sta-bilizing so that expansion can hold within you. Use the complete session each day with extended times for Head Position #3 and Front Positions #1 and #3.*[5]

Journeying with Light

The following sharing by Sue Maxwell first appeared in *Living in Radiance*, a journal of The Radiance Technique Association for Great Britain. When Sue was diagnosed with cancer, she had only recently taken The Second Degree. She went on to study The Radiant Third Degree and used TRT® as a support throughout the process. She wrote this, sharing

15 months on from the first prognosis, which had measured her life in months. Sue actually lived a full three years with an expanded quality of life, continuing to grow and transform as a human being. She made her transition naturally and peacefully, and when the moment came, quickly in July 1998, family and friends using The Radiance Technique® Hands-on as well as the inner-planes networking of many directing Radiant energy and Attunements supported her. Those who knew her treasure her passion for living, her radiant persistence, joy and commitment to others. Sue's whole life was a celebration of our human journey.

"On the eve of my 50th birthday in August 1995, my little world stopped turning. What appeared to be a mild mastitis masked a particularly virulent form of breast cancer. It was the worst grade measurable, invasive and fast growing. Immediate surgery was prescribed either as a radical mastectomy with all underarm glands removed or partial removal with chemotherapy. In either case, radiotherapy would be required.

"I have lived my life gently along holistic guidelines as a life-vegetarian, and I am a practicing herbalist. I was unused to drugs of any chemical type. I did not believe that one could 'cut out' a disease. Yet, everyone whose opinion I respected told me that this was a very serious situation and that to stand a chance I had to 'do everything.' I opted for partial surgery with chemotherapy in order to retain use of my arm for my massage work.

"Immediate surgery revealed that the cancer had spread into the lymph glands and was passing through a duct wall into the bloodstream. I was not told quite how little time I was estimated to have, but I wasn't expected to see Christmas.

"My plan was to pursue every natural means possible of coping with cancer, explore the roots of my own case with inner work, try to live a semblance of normal life and confront the fact I had a real imbalance of immunity when I thought I was living a rich and pretty fulfilling life.

"Two weeks to the day of surgery, I gave my first full body massage. Normal assessment for physiotherapy is three months. One month later, I started chemotherapy. Normally, this can now be balanceable, allowing patients to live relatively normal lives. But because my cancer was so serious and because there was a major unknown factor, my experience was violent. The body that was totally unused to chemical drugs reacted to the poison and the support drugs. I hallucinated, lost my sight, developed tinnitus, vomited and shook. My skin fell off and my heart raced. I felt as if a team of wild horses was pulling me apart. After a month, the specialist was not sure I would be strong enough to endure the course of chemotherapy.

"The whole thing threw me into an inner place, a land of nightmares. With the aid of acupuncture, herbs, healing foods and lots of energy work, my symptoms came under control. Here it was that I was able to use The Radiance Technique. The simple, effortless, hands-on opened up a depth of healing/wholing power that enhanced all my natural support systems. I was able to use TRT® to transmute that darkness into Light.

"By now, I had been working with TRT® for four years and The Second Degree for three years. I had used it daily in the course of my work but less frequently on myself. Now I had the incentive to give myself daily sessions. When I was capable of nothing else, I could place my hands in a position and drift into my Cosmic Symbols. Often a peaceful sleep would follow, and I would awaken later with my hands still in place, body rhythms settling. The positivity and energy that filled me would push away the darkness and a feeling of being connected would replace the isolation and loneliness that the impaired senses had given me.

"I had been used to practicing TRT® on other people and had been conscious that giving it directly to myself had not been a priority. This is just one of the many things I have learned during my adventure with breast cancer. It's a lesson that I might never have otherwise learned, for 'giving to myself' had been difficult for me.

"I also held my medication and patterned the Cosmic Symbols over it, visualizing the heavy drugs transforming into light medicine and used the same process to vitalize my food.

"Through a very dark winter, I managed to complete the full chemotherapy course. There were times when I was strong enough to continue my work, and patients reported enthusiastically there was an added significance to my hands-on work and that the treatments were deeper and more profound. The rest of the time, my senses were so impaired, social isolation prevailed as family grieved and dealt with their shock, and close friends, in some cases, withdrew to deal with the situation. They feared if it could happen to me, with my way of life — then it could happen to them.

"On a physical level, I still felt battered, but people around me sensed my energy levels as vibrant, positive and glowing all the time. I lived mostly with a humour and lightness that transformed what could have been an unbearably dark experience. I was drawn to positive people and enjoyed spending time on my own. I avoided people with negative outlooks, for they only seemed to drain my energies.

"Often, I would be conscious of the uplifting energies that were being directed to me, the thoughts and prayers of so many people — asking for nothing in return — that seemed to hold a great net of love around me. Of the people whom I was conscious of sending me help, my TRT® teacher, Ingrid St. Clare, was very important to me. Many times, I was conscious of her support, and believed it was, and continues to be, invaluable. She continued to direct Radiant energy for me regularly, and when she was able to reach me, she gave me hands-on sessions that were beautiful and profound. At times, my body lit up like neon!

"The end of the chemotherapy arrived to much jubilation on the part of the specialists. I had not grown any further tumours. I was congratulated for enduring it and sent off to prepare for the radiotherapy. Within an hour, a routine scan told another story. No one had checked my liver. Each specialist had thought the other had checked. The chemotherapy drugs they had used were useless. It was now too late to have any treatment at all. I had to go home and prepare my family with the news that I had approximately three weeks to live.

"I tried to believe it. Everyone was in agreement. Yet, I had no sense of impending death. Faith in my intuition was shattered. How could I be so out of touch with myself? For two weeks, I tried to get my head around preparations for death and then stopped. My intuition was telling me I would not die now. However foolish it seemed to others, I had to be true to myself and I threw myself into living positively with the natural support therapies and TRT®.

"The specialist did not expect to see me again. Two months later, at an appointment he explained was made to humour me, his jaw fell as he saw me in the waiting room. I was swimming again and working more. The very rapid form must have been slowing down. Some of the tumours must have been dying. This was not something he had met before or seen documented at such an advanced stage of terminal illness.

"The adventure continues; I explore and research every natural treatment that I can access, but the core of my process is TRT® energy work. I have ups and downs, and there have been times that I have felt like a close call. Often, my body has declined even herbs as too caustic and struggled with acidic fruits, but the energy of TRT® is always possible. Since it is technically impossible, they tell me, for my body to be functioning so normally, I attribute it to the fact that on an energy level, I am being fully and vibrantly supported. I have no jaundice, my quality of life is good, and my digestion is excellent. I have only minor distension and inflammation; my pain level is exceptionally low whereas I would be expected to need two whole grams of morphine a day. And I am still working.

"Of course, there needs to be a lot of time invested in caring for my body, including concern with food, getting enough rest and not overdoing things. TRT® is central to the rest periods and the energizing of my food. Patterning the cosmic spiral is so automatic in my life now that I barely notice doing it. Increasingly, I realize it is the energy work that I am drawn to and benefitting from. Towards the end of last year, it was possible for me to do The Radiant Third Degree. This meant an enormous amount to me and proved to be a profound experience. The new vibration was smoother and seemed to have an extra dimension.

"One whole year on from the day of my 'death sentence,' I stood on top of the Grand Canyon, fulfilling a life's ambition. To get there, I'd endured three thousand miles and three weeks of changing altitude, different beds, snow, ice and heat. This was a far different experience than the one I was expected to have. My journey culminated in Sedona, Arizona, where huge red rocks, each with its own power vortex, tower majestically upwards from sacred lands. Conscious of the power, many therapists work here and many people come for healing, but I felt no need for outside help. Gradually, the pulling and tugging that I could sense so strongly began to settle into a new rhythm. I knew that TRT® would embrace it all.

"Fifteen months later, my personal journey continues. My specialist is incredulous that I am still here. My Macmillan Nurse no longer talks of the hospice. Visitors say our home is vibrant with energy. My patients claim to gain more benefit from sessions than ever, and it is difficult to see my adventure with cancer as anything other than a profound and positive learning. Technically, it is not possible for my body to function, but it does and I believe it is doing this on an energy level. The energy work becomes more important to me all the time and is always appropriate.

"'Whatever you are doing,' says my specialist, 'continue — and don't let anyone intervene because you have broken new ground and achieved something that could not be envisaged as possible, something beyond anything we could have imagined.' Life is not always easy; it needs constant focus and flexibility, but my sense is that I am fully alive. I feel like a healthy person in the middle of a great adventure, with so much still to learn and so much still to do. I perceive that anything is possible on an energy level where perhaps my own healing has also taken place. Whether it has or not, with The Radiance Technique®, I continue to celebrate being fully alive in every sense."[6]

People over and over again comment on how TRT® contributes and supports a higher quality of life. As Dr. Barbara Ray writes:

> *Quality of Life — Regardless of your age, occupation and/ or personal interests, one of the most important aspects of wholeness and wellness is the <u>quality</u> of your life. Your life is an unfolding, a process of discovery and a journey within which you can awaken to the multi-dimensions of yourself. No matter what challenges you may be experiencing on any level of your energy dimensions, you can begin now to appreciate and to honor your life energy as a growing and transforming person. Daily applications of The Radiance Technique® give you the opportunity to access <u>directly</u> and <u>for yourself</u> radiant, universal transcendental energy which expands and enhances the quality of your experience of life.[7]*

Life Energy Connection for Chronic Fatigue

Debra Farrer is a wife and mother of two young adults in their 20s. She has been married for over 26 years to her husband who was also her childhood friend. Debra was a registered nurse for many years before her collision with CFIDS and fibromyalgia. She shares her journey in the following:

"Before beginning TRT®, I rarely left my home. Any venture outside of my home, where I kept as calm, quiet and low stimulating an environment as possible exacerbated all of my symptoms to an even greater debilitating state. Even to have someone come into my home was added stimulation that would cause the same reaction. Physically, emotionally and mentally, I was constantly struggling to just get through the days.

In October 2001, I found my way to The First Degree Official Program of The Radiance Technique®, Authentic Reiki®. Immediately, I was aware of the healing nature of TRT® and by the 16th day of hands-on, I experienced a number of life-changing epiphanies. I continued daily doing more than a full one hour session, as I knew that I had finally found the key to unlocking not only the chains of my illness, but the weight that I carried with me throughout life. The results have been what can only be described as a miracle of healing. I began exercising, using the same muscles that over the past 15 years tolerated so very little, without exhaustion, of not only physical energy but also mental clarity and emotional stability.

"Now, I feel a life energy in me that seems to have no limits. I have an energy that is not only stronger but one that is thriving and growing on a daily basis. I have a life force energy on all levels that has taken me to a place I had no expectation of embracing when I first set out on my journey with TRT®. Two years later, I took The Second Degree and I enjoy the flexibility it has given me. I incorporate the symbols in all aspects of my life including driving long distances. I like the fact that I can direct to people I know who are in need, people who live far from me, or near, and they don't need to be aware that I am directing this Radiant light energy to them. Overall, I feel much more connected to others than I have ever been in my life.

"I look back on my physical energy which used to rate a 3 or 4 out of 10 on a day to day average. Now my days are an average of 6 to 8 out of 10, with many days on a level of an 8 or better. There are still days of recuperation after much physical labour, but I am able to work at a pace that I have not known for over 17 years. And my time spent in recuperation has significantly decreased. Of all my symptoms, the change in my energy level is the one that is most dramatically noticeable.

"What I have come to know so far is this: I am becoming more fully aware of my growth and expansion, and have noticed a huge paradigm shift both emotionally and mentally. What were once huge struggles in the past, causing stress and anxiety, I now see in a very different light and with a calm acceptance. I no longer feel the need to control that which I cannot control, especially when it comes to other people and their nature to be who they are.

"As my thinking becomes less rigid, especially with regards to others, I have seen and experienced unlimited possibilities for myself, such as greater peace within, a stronger sense of self-esteem, and confidence in who I am. I do not depend on the actions or words of others to support my own sense of self, especially from those who are not capable of doing so. I feel less stress and anxiety when interacting with these same individuals, and I am now seeing a change in how they interact with me! I have seen that I am now able to love these same individuals, from my heart centre, with unconditional love! In the past, my feelings of hurt, frustration and anger were huge barriers to loving and accepting them. I have seen the resentment of many years fall by the wayside, allowing a greater sense of peace within. I find that I am also experiencing unconditional love for others in general. I experience greater clarity of thought and, with that, an awareness of connecting to my inner wisdom. I am experiencing universal awakening!

"I know that I will continue to be transformed daily with the use of TRT®and can see no limit to its incredible power to change not only my wholeness, but of course my life in the process. As I transform and see the changes in my life, the more I am inspired to use TRT®not only for myself, but for the support of all light energy of our planet.

"I have been often told that I sound like a different person over the phone, and that I look like a different person in appearance! Few people know what it is I am doing differently these days, but when I can, I share with them the gift and power of TRT®in my life. I am practicing the art of *living Radiantly in the moment* and that brings me great peace."

Healing through Meningitis and Encephalitis

My good friend Marina Linardou of Athens, Greece, has been living with her life-threatening illness for nine years now. As a wife, mother and former teacher she still has days when normal, every day activities are challenging. She has studied to The Fourth Degree and received her first introduction to The Radiance Technique® 15 years ago. Her story begins with her journey to the hospital.

"On January 7th, 1997, an ambulance took me to the hospital," she explains. "The first diagnosis was an infection from a virus and sinusitis. Somehow, I knew that the diagnosis was incorrect, and I was suspecting meningitis, but the doctors did not believe me. I was getting worse and worse. I started to lose my ability to move. Gradually, I lost my sight and hearing, and repeated seizures blocked my breathing. Finally, the analysis of the cerebral spinal liquid gave a correct diagnosis: meningitis-encephalitis from the bacteria pneumoniococus. I was in a coma for several days and the prognosis was not good. During these critical days of my illness, my mother, who had The Second Degree, called friends who had studied

The Radiance Technique® and together they directed Radiant energy. My mother believed that I was close to making my transition. Today she thinks the fact I am alive and healthy is due to a miracle!

"It took me a long time to recover. This was a very hard and painful period with lots of complications. During my hospitalization and afterwards, TRT® has always been there to support me. It has been my precious tool for the difficult moments, when I was completely alone with my pain both on a physical and psychological level. The Radiant TRT Heart First Ashram® Healing/Wholing Network opened its 'doors' to let me in, and embraced and held me in a huge Radiant hug in this journey towards my fulfillment and enlightenment.

"Before I studied TRT®, I had attended many different seminars that were meant to expand my knowledge and help me come closer to finding my real self. From the very first moment of my class in The First Degree Official Program of The Radiance Technique®, Authentic Reiki®, I knew deep in my heart that I had finally found what I was looking for all these years of studying, searching and questioning. I feel grateful to my teacher Barbara Aurora for being a Radiant expression of her teachings and for giving me this precious and unique tool to use anytime, anywhere and everywhere.

"I continue to use TRT® in many different ways: hands-on, symbols and attunements. It has become a way of life, a source of joy, a healing, wholing experience for my health, for my family, and for ongoing day-to-day challenges. After some years of study, it was enough just to envision my hands on my heart centre, or envision one of the Cosmic Symbols, or hear the whisper of the words *The Radiant TRT Heart First Ashram®*, to feel the inner connection between me and all the other beings around the world. What an incredible joy, support and expansion. And every time was different and deeper, on a different level of consciousness, but always more profound and expansive. An experience of healing that comes from within, not only on a physical, psychological or spiritual level, but a profound healing experience on all levels. Healing is a process that has no beginning or end, it is just healing and wholing from within forever."

Surviving and Thriving

In the summer of 1994, Christa Naeckel was in her 18th year of driving a bus for Windsor Transit when she received news of her diagnosis. She had a large tumour on her upper left lip that turned out to be adenoid cystic carcinoma of the minor salivary gland, a very rare type of cancer. Her surgeon told her it was incurable and that she had six months to live. She remembers that moment well:

"When the doctor told me, I was lying on the stretcher. I froze. I was white like a sheet and I could not drive. The nurse had to bring me home. So many things went through my mind. I cried a lot and had an anxiety attack.

"I had to wait two more months for a second surgery. Radiation therapy was recommended, as the doctors did not get all of the cancer during surgery. The initial treatments were difficult, for I could not focus or remember things. I couldn't eat and I had trouble speaking; I was a vegetable. I called my friend who suggested I contact Hospice for support. I saw a nurse and social worker there that referred me to Radiant Touch®.

"I was the type of person who was skeptical at first. I was not sure if this was going to work but knew that I could not lose. The first time I went to a Radiant Touch® session it was okay, the second time it was okay, and the third time I noticed that I really relaxed and I felt good. I could not feel my arms or head. Everything was just floating.

"After my third session, I drove to the hospital for my radiation treatment. When they pinned me to the table with a mask over my face, they could do anything with me because I was so light, like pudding. My TRT® sessions made my body more responsive to the radiation and medical treatments.

"Gradually my attitude began to change. Whenever I went to the hospital for my treatments, I did not cry or remain in a depressed mood. In fact, I cheered a lot of other people up. I had always been a people person, doing for others, but never relied on having others do for me. I could not believe the support I received, and I learned to allow people to help me too.

"I continued Radiant Touch® sessions and became more proactive in my care. I listened to relaxation tapes between my sessions. I focused on good nutrition for my body. During radiation treatments, I took supplement drinks like Ensure and when I could eat again, I cooked fresher foods.

"Six months later, I studied The First Degree Official Program of The Radiance Technique®, Authentic Reiki®, and I loved the fact that I could do it for myself every day. When I was stressed, I used especially Head Positions #1-3 and this helped with headache pain.

"When I completed radiation, the doctor asked me what I did, considering I was always so cheerful and tolerated things so well. You would have never thought that I had only six months to live. I was so grateful for the wonderful care and support I received. My recovery and my well-being are due to the combination of the radiation, the surgery, my TRT® sessions, my thoughts and my diet. Now ten years later, I am still here and doctors can't believe it!

"I have faced death and I see life differently. There are a lot of things that used to be very important to me — material things are not as important. What is important for me is my well-being, my three children and my four grandchildren. I treasure the little things and my family, and I'm so happy that I am still here. I feel good. I find that I am more in tune with my body; my body tells me what I need. In the past, I went like a robot, reacting to stress and just kept going, no matter what. I feel healthy with no pain anywhere. My sinus problems and headaches have disappeared. I live day by day and every day is special. TRT® has helped my quality of life and has been an important part of my healing journey. Wherever I go, I always have my radiant hands."

Living Life Fully with Lung Cancer

Sandra Chase-Ellwood, R.N., lived her life to its fullest. Despite the odds of her prognosis, she married a wonderful husband, bought a house, had a beautiful daughter and participated in the May '98 Hospice 10-km walk. She had been diagnosed three years earlier with an inoperable form of lung cancer. She was on the front page of The Windsor Star newspaper with her nine-month-old daughter Iesha. The paper wrote, "Her cancer can't be easily explained — she never smoked, nor does she have a family history of lung cancer: The future for most lung cancer patients is not bright. Of approximately 330 local people who get it each year; only 15 per cent are alive after five years. But Chase continues to beat the odds and believes she will conquer her cancer."[8]

From the first moment we met, Sandra and I had a special connection. We had both experienced cancer and were approximately the same age, but it was more than that. We shared intimate talks about life, our purpose, our hopes, our cooking and music. Each time I saw her, I was in awe of this incredible woman with an amazing spirit. Despite her daughter's challenges connected to Down's syndrome, Sandra displayed incredible strength, resilience and limitless love. She was an active parent to her daughter from day one. She worked hard to bring family together and was instrumental in a lot of family healing. She gave me many gifts, the greatest one being gratitude. Gratitude to live life to the fullest — to share, to laugh, to cry, to be real and in the moment. Anyone who met her was transformed by her tenacity to keep going. Her prognosis was not good, but she always had hope for cure. She made her transition on December 11, 2000, five years after her initial diagnosis. Sandra wrote and shared the following with me in 1998 and 1999:

"I always believed that there were 'forces' to keep one well. Soon after my diagnosis, I sought out the support of Hospice and I was referred for sessions of TRT®. During the sessions, I went to a cloud; it was really peaceful for me. TRT® was giving me peace; I was not as worried, not as tense. It brought me on a road of peacefulness and to me, peacefulness is health. I decided to take The First Degree Official Program of The Radiance Technique®, Authentic Reiki®. TRT® gave me flexibility; I could do it when I needed it.

"There are a number of techniques that I use to stay healthy mentally, physically, emotionally and spiritually, and TRT® helps me to attain and maintain a high level of health. I use TRT® everyday. It's become part of my life just like praying, eating and sleeping but it's not quite routine. I might do full body TRT® two to three times a week, and whenever I do this, I always fall asleep. I set my watch to beep every five minutes so I know when to change positions. Now a full session should take 1 hour, but for me, it is always 1 hour and 20 minutes or more so I know somewhere in that session I must have fallen asleep, but I don't know where. I always wake up feeling recharged. If I have a nap during the day, I often wake up feeling worse than when I laid down, but not when I use TRT®.

"Sometimes, I use Head Positions #1, #2, #3 and #4 before I get out of bed in the morning. I really find that even doing Head Positions #1 and #2 before I get out of bed opens up my sinuses. I can feel them drain into the back of my throat. This is great because before TRT®, I would feel fine; I didn't even realize that my sinuses were slightly plugged.

"And everyday, my favourite position is Front Position #2. I do this watching TV, at the doctor's office, in church. I find this position very relaxing. It helps me to focus on what's going on in front of me or what is being said. I don't sleep on my back, but if I do this position in bed while flat on my back, feet slightly apart, I become so relaxed I'm asleep in five minutes.

"I don't actually have to think about it. I do TRT® all the time when I have chest pain, neck pain or jaw pain. It is automatic. It helps with my pain. It brings me to a spot where I don't think about the pain.

"When you have pain, all your senses are on. I have pain; TRT® brings me to a place where I don't think about the pain. My energy level fluctuates; my breathing fluctuates. I do TRT® first, and then I go for the groceries or any other shopping.

"During my pregnancy, I used hands-on to support me and calm me. Iesha is such a good and happy baby. While breast-feeding, I use hands-on. She was baby Jesus in church one Christmas, up in the manger alone for one hour, and she did not cry. She also received Attunements for The First Degree Official Program of The Radiance Technique®, Authentic Reiki®.

"I mainly do TRT® because I believe it helps to balance the energies in my body so my body is better able to use its energy to fight off the cancer cells that it is dealing with instead of fighting stress, emotional distress, fatigue and sometimes pain. I feel that the absence of the mental chitter chatter, the peace, the energy that I feel after doing TRT® is all just a bonus. I was diagnosed with lung cancer three and a half years ago, and through the grace of God and my wellness program, which includes TRT® daily, I'm still here."

Self-Care During Colon Cancer

Kveta was diagnosed in the spring of 1997 with colon cancer that had spread to her liver and urethra. She immigrated to

Canada from Slovakia in 1995 and admits working two jobs with long hours, no vacation and no relaxation. Her recent divorce caused her much stress, and she was left alone to take care of herself. The news of diagnosis caused Kveta to change her life on all levels.

"After recovering from the shock and then the cancer operation, I started looking for some kind of help. Feeling that there must be more than chemotherapy and radiation, which I went through without success, I turned my attention to Hospice. It was the best step I could have taken. I met extraordinary people there having understanding and compassion. One of the services I used was TRT®. Each session for me had been like a light in the tunnel. During hands-on, I felt a surge of energy, experienced optimism and hope for surviving. Each time, I walked away relaxed, peaceful and stronger to deal with my fate.

"I soon learned The First Degree Official Program of The Radiance Technique®, Authentic Reiki®, and I could give myself hands-on whenever I felt anxious or stressed. Getting a diagnosis like I did forces you to look at your life, forces you to live and changes your perception. I have never been so focused on my body in my life, taking care and nurturing it."

As time progressed, Kveta received an operation for a colostomy, and she became more conscious of what she ate. TRT®became integrated into her life. She employed Radiant Touch®for meditation, during prayer, during yoga and exercises, while cooking her food and while holding her medication and vitamins. She was using it every day in every way.

Kveta felt some of her friends did not really understand what she was going through. "One friend told me that she is booking her appointment to get her eyes lifted while another just finished a whole face lift and liposuction," she says, "and here I am planning my funeral."

Her ankles increasingly began to swell, she retained more

fluids, and her kidneys began to shut down. It became more and more difficult to walk up the two flights of stairs to her apartment to carry groceries. She rarely left her apartment, which became her haven of peace, warmly decorated with pictures from home on vibrantly coloured painted walls. Kveta expressed how her body felt like a stranger within her. She experienced a change in her appetite and increased difficulty in swallowing. She encountered more constipation and more pain. She was working closely with her physician for pain control. "I was on Tylenol #3 two weeks ago and now I am on morphine. However, even though I feel as weak as I do, I can still do some of the TRT® positions. I feel 'Wow,' I did something good for me; it is like giving myself hope and peace. I have learned a lot lately about my body. Holding my hands in certain positions for a longer period of time composes my body, and I feel better. With Front Position #4, I feel a lot of relief. I feel strength here too. Now I know why people call Dr. Kervorkian; I experienced unbearable pain before I began the morphine. My connection to my spirit is what is keeping me going. When I do hands-on, I connect to my spiritual self. It is like 'going home.' I feel immersed, like I am really with me and God and in relationship with Him because physically I have to say..." and she closed her eyes and tears began.

During one of our sessions, Kveta had a vision to go home, back to Slovakia for Christmas. The miracles began. She received a free flight from her colleagues at work, and her daughter rearranged her wedding to coincide with the time of Kveta's arrival. She had shared with me that she felt like she was at the end of her journey but would go home one last time. We increased our hands-on sessions and the physician worked with her to have all her medication in place. The whole thing was a miracle. I remember seeing her before she left and helped her pack her things. It was a joyous, timeless moment.

After attending her daughter's wedding and celebrating the holidays, Kveta made her transition surrounded by her family and grandchildren in the town where she was born.

Help for People Living with AIDS

A groundbreaking book written by Van Ault blazed the way of documenting the quiet support TRT®has given to people living with AIDS. In *The Radiance Technique® and AIDS,* Van reveals his discoveries, challenges and personal experiences using TRT®. His unique perspective provides inspiration for those facing an AIDS diagnosis:

"The challenges of AIDS are many. While the disease has struck a harsh blow to especially vulnerable populations, it has motivated many of us to contemplate a broader spectrum of responses and options. It has also compelled us to fully claim the power of choice in our health-care decisions. The choice to nurture ourselves, the choice to explore new, joyous dimensions of life, and the choice to actively express our whole selves — not just our personalities — are all supported by The Radiance Technique®.

"TRT® certainly has opened up more choices for those of us committed to applying Radiant energy in our lives. For the people whose sharings are included in this book, practicing this technique has been nurturing and empowering in ways that no social service, political activism or other external effort could hope to be. TRT® invites a transformation that begins in the centre of our consciousness and then unfolds harmoniously into our physical, mental and emotional realms. ...

"The Radiance Technique® offers us direct access to an impersonal, transpersonal source of inner compassion. The energy it supplies is not limited by overwhelming outer circumstances, and one can draw upon it in any situation. That energy can enhance our quality of life substantially, an essential factor in this health holocaust. For many of us with HIV, it is not enough simply to survive the epidemic if there is nothing more for us than to endure its starkness. We want to survive and *thrive*, with a high *quality of life* that makes our physical existence worth preserving, exploring, and celebrating."[9]

Van's contribution to people living with AIDS inspired Marcia Ward to wish to help others. Marcia first studied TRT® in 1982 and found that it changed her quality of life. She has many chronic health conditions, and despite them all, she has been able to use and support others with Radiant Touch® at The North Winds Living Centre in Oklahoma City, USA. Marcia is an Authorized Instructor with The Seventh Degree.

"I suffer from hypertension, fibromyalgia, degenerative disc disease in my neck, chronic fatigue and cataracts," she says. "The older I get, the more parts of my physical body break down. Through my years of study with TRT®, I am learning to nurture the part of me that has more permanence than the parts of me that are impermanent.

"I can see past the pain of the patients that I work with. I can see past their lifestyles. And I can see the love within them. I can accept their transitions more easily and see the process for what it is — natural. I feel that this acceptance I have of them and whom they really are enables both of us to share love of the highest nature.

"I have been a volunteer at North Winds since 1996. People living with AIDS live in a home-like, non-judgemental environment, which offers a life filled with dignity and love. When I first started working on the patients, I would go into their rooms, use a stool and ask them if anything hurt. Then a few months later, I brought in a table for the sessions. Each patient who wished to receive TRT®also received the attunements of The First Degree, and I often put them on the The Radiant TRT Heart First Ashram® Healing/Wholing Network for support. I would like to share a few of my experiences with very special people.

"My first patient was Paula who was in her early 40s. She

wanted TRT®right away. She was in a wheel chair and went for dialysis three times a week due to kidney failure. I always used TRT®on the shunt in her arm as well as complete an entire session with her. For her neuropathy, I gave her attunements on her feet and spiral massages on her legs. I massaged gently with cream and my Radiant hands. I gave her an Attunement and showed her how to massage it for herself. The neuropathy seemed to slow down when the legs and feet had some circulation. It was after this she began walking.

"Paula was a hard worker and used TRT®on herself daily. Her viral load became undetectable. Soon she was working with a physical therapist and walking short distances. By the next year, she was marching in AIDS parades. She had periodic visits to the hospital because the blood pressure could not be corrected for a length of time. They never had to relocate her shunt the entire time she was working with TRT®.

"A year from our first meeting, Paula moved out of North Winds into her own apartment in assisted living. Although she died two years later, she had an improved quality of life since using The Radiance Technique®.

"An amazing experience documenting the power of directing Radiant energy from all over the world is my experience with Kevin. One winter morning he fell and broke his jaw. Due to his age, 58, and the fact that he had HIV, the doctor had to remove all of his lower teeth and put in a steel plate from side to side. He was in a great amount of pain and moved in and out of the hospital awaiting surgery. I decided to submit his name to the TRTIA Healing/Wholing Network. When it was first sent, his T-cell count was 12. Kevin's count is now over 500.

"When I first met Bill, he was still in shock after learning that he had AIDS. He apparently contacted the virus through a blood transfusion years before. A local hospital misdiagnosed him as having TB, and the resulting treatment caused the AIDS to manifest.

"When he came to the North Winds, he was depressed and ill with congestive heart failure and severe neuropathy. The circulation in his legs was so bad that they were turning black. Bill was a Shrine Clown and made balloon animals for other patients. He was friendly and kind to all. After reading our handout on TRT® that we give to all new patients, he was eager for a session on the table.

"Bill had a profound experience with TRT®. Whenever he was well enough, he would come for hands-on. At times, he could even walk down the hall to us.

"A few months passed and I witnessed his rapid decline. Towards the end, he knew I was doing hands-on and he joined me by putting his hands on top of mine, guiding my hands to where he wanted them, where he had pain and discomfort. Within those three weeks, he passed on.

"Another patient who I had a special connection with was John. At the time he was in his 50s and complaining of neuropathy in his feet. He responded well to my hands on his feet. I would spend a half hour to one hour holding his feet and using cosmic symbols and Attunements.

"As time went on and he got used to me, I began the complete hands-on session. Every few weeks we would alternate: feet one week and then entire body. He complained about depression and this often set in immediately after a fellow patient made his/her transition. John had been at North Winds since it opened. His mother had died there just down the hall during the first year of its operation.

"After supporting John for a few months of complete sessions, he began to use his hands upon himself and this became a regular part of his own self-care. He was instrumental in getting other patients to try TRT®.

"As time went on, John began to make dream catchers and woven bracelets. His attitude began to improve and he began sharing his crafts with others and sometimes even teaching them. He helped plant and tend a garden of vegetables, an activity that was very healing for him.

"A year later during the fall, John found lumps below his right breast and on the top of his head. He had them removed and discovered they were cancerous. Soon there were lumps all over his head and torso. I listed his first name on the TRTIA Healing/Wholing Network for directed Radiant energy support. With each update, he seemed to be more accepting of his upcoming transition. I decorated his door and we called it The Gateway. He made his transition in the early spring.

"And I will never forget the transition of Jack. He was a tiny man who came from a family of farmers and was very ill. His acceptance of TRT® opened a gateway for him. He shared with me that through the hands-on sessions he felt he 'was receiving love.'

"I am filled with gratitude to be a support and guide to people on their journey. I have noticed that people who have a good attitude, take their medication and receive Radiant energy support experience healing shifts, whether they remain on the physical plane or transit to another."

[1] Katherine Lenel, *The Radiance Technique® and Cancer*, (St. Petersburg, FL: Radiance Associates, 1994), p. 20.

[2] *Ibid.*

[3] Ray, *The Expanded Reference Manual of The Radiance Technique®, Authentic Reiki®*, p. 115.

[4] Canadian Cancer Society/National Cancer Institute of Canada: *Canadian Cancer Statistics 2007*, Toronto, Canada, 2007. p. 20.

[5] Ray, *The Expanded Reference Manual of The Radiance Technique®, Authentic Reiki®*, p. 92.

[6] Sue Maxwell, 'Journeying with Light-a personal account of coping with cancer,' *Living in Radiance*, Issue One, The Radiance Technique Association for Great Britain, 1997, p. 8.

[7] Ray, *The Expanded Reference Manual of The Radiance Technique®, Authentic Reiki®*, p. 91.

[8] 'Hospice fundraising walk rekindles hope, memories,' by Brian Cross, *The Windsor Star*, May 16, 1998, p. A1.

[9] Van Ault, *The Radiance Technique® and AIDS*, (San Francisco, CA: Resources for Renewal, 1996), p. 107.

PART 3

Unveiling

Consciously pausing life's revolving demands,
Restoring balance through Radiant hands.

Letting go of the turmoil that festers within,
Unleashing inner energy so healing may begin.

Like a drop of water becomes part of the sea,
Connecting to the universe to fulfill our destiny.

Expanding our vision to see through new eyes,
Relishing each moment, persevering through hard times.

Nurturing our entire mind, body and soul,
Loving not certain parts, but honouring our whole.

A state of deep relaxation and quieting the mind,
Discovering new paths, priceless treasures we will find.

Pure white light reaches every corner of our being,
As each atom surrenders, it operates with new meaning.

The endless comparison to be like someone else,
Learning true serenity is to be true to yourself.

Starting with self-love we will find genuine tranquility,
Choosing to be grateful, we must give unconditionally.

Centring ourselves using our values as our guide,
Feeling our inner strength and security not to hide.

As an artist paints expressing their creativity,
So do I unveil a new layer of my authenticity.

~ Christa Papineau, Caregiver

Caregivers Along the Way

"I have used Radiant Touch® with my father who is living with cancer. It is with thankfulness and privilege that I can support him in affirming his wish and want for a better quality of life and well-being.

~ *Linda Sabatini*
Hospice Service Coordinator

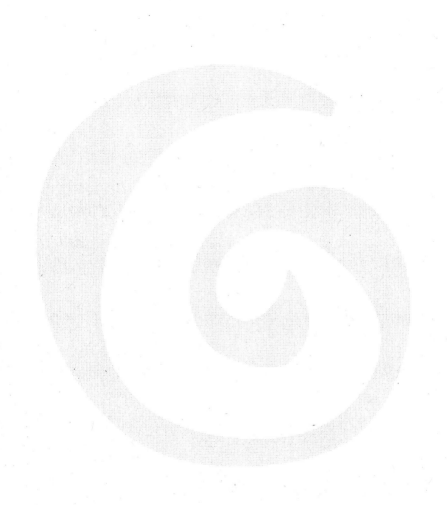

-4-

WHEN SOMEONE CLOSE TO US IS DIAGNOSED with a life-threatening illness, one of the greatest challenges is how we will respond to them. The news touches us deeply inside, to the core of our being. It often involves struggles within our mind and heart and its emotional nature. We want to do everything in our power to help. Illness affects the entire family — spouse, children, sisters, brothers, neighbours, colleagues, close friends and pets. It is an intense and intimate experience. The Radiance Technique® supports the caregiver's resilience and quest for balance during these challenges.

Home Care Movement

We have witnessed a new form of caregiving outside the traditional institution walls. The movement for home care in Canada expanded in the late 1980s due to budget constraints, and hospital cutbacks. This shift caused family members to be more directly involved in caring for someone at home. Families are faced with a multitude of responsibilities including learning new health care lingo, giving medications and scheduling their life around professional caregivers coming to the home. The dilemma of making decisions about medical life-prolonging procedures, such as artificial hydration and nutrition, resuscitation and ventilator support, adds to the stress. This can lead to deep struggles within that accompany such choices. Concern about the receiver's quality of care, his or her dignity and quality of life are the focus. Family caregivers are on duty

24 hours a day and are often tired and stressed. Furthermore, critics claim that these symptoms are increasing: "Even before the most recent cutbacks in service, research indicated that caregivers have higher rates of depressive and anxiety disorders and use mental health services twice as much. Older, unpaid caregivers reported increased stress, high blood pressure, exhaustion, and susceptibility to physical illness."[1]

Providing care and support for another individual is demanding. It can last for weeks, months or even years. One's life changes as the challenges of ongoing daily responsibilities of caregiving are added to work, raising a family and personal care. And if we look around, we will see primarily women shoulder that caregiving. According to one authority, "estimates indicate that around 90% of health care is provided at home by unpaid providers, indicating that women in particular are carrying heavy caring workloads along with their paid jobs."[2] Often, the basics like nutrition, exercise and adequate sleep suffer. Caregivers find themselves lacking energy and having short tempers. No time for themselves highlights the many thoughts running back and forth in their mind. Many express feeling overwhelmed, riding an emotional roller coaster of feeling angry one minute, guilty the next and depressed all at the same time. In many cases, feelings of helplessness, inadequacy or failure frequently prevail. I have witnessed more caregivers burned out while providing care, and they were not even aware of it because all of it became "normal" in their everyday lives. Their reservoir of energy continuously depletes with no means of filling it up.

However, convincing caregivers to care for themselves is one of the biggest challenges facing hospices. The two common themes heard all the time are *I can't leave his/her side* and *I feel guilty if I take time for me*. And it is not easy to change the attitudes and beliefs a caregiver might have. For some, they don't know how to give care for themselves, and others believe that they don't matter — family is first and foremost.

Some worry about what others would think; their expectations, beliefs and culture play a role as well. Learn to recognize the warning signs of stress through the following checklist.

Caregiver Stress Signs and Symptoms

Stress affects the physical, emotional, mental and behavioural parts of you and is not always the same for each person. If you are a caregiver, you should look for help from a local support group, health agency or counsellor if you are experiencing some of the following:

Emotional
- You feel overwhelmed and pressured. No matter what you do, it doesn't seem to be enough.
- You feel depressed. It feels like there are no more happy times.
- You feel alone and isolated.
- You don't feel loving and caring like you used to.
- You are becoming argumentative, short tempered.
- You feel like crying.
- Despite all your caregiving, your loved one is still getting worse.

Mental
- You have difficulty remembering things.
- You find you are more negative than your usual self.
- You feel like you can't stop the racing thoughts in your mind.

Physical
- You have trouble sleeping or feel like sleeping all the time.
- You experience shortness of breath or have difficulty catching your breath.
- You have increased pain.
- You feel exhausted.

Behavioural
- Your coping methods have become destructive: you're overeating or under eating, you are increasing your use of tobacco, alcohol, drugs, or medications.
- You feel it's selfish to ever think of yourself or your needs at this time.
- You feel your relationships with others are suffering because of all the pressure.

We all begin with the best intentions, but lengthy illnesses, lack of support and constant exposure to those who are suffering can lead us to feel overwhelmed and exhausted. This applies to family, friends, and volunteers, as well as professional caregivers. The stress arising from overload can lead to insensitivity, depression and feelings of helplessness. The inability to recognize and respond to signs and symptoms of stress will lead to burn out. On this subject, Dr. Barbara Ray offers the following:

> *"**Burn Out**" — Refers to physical, emotional and/or mental exhaustion from long-term stress. Often the exhaustion is accompanied by feelings of being overwhelmed, or observing a lack of creativity or zest for the work at hand. The daily and ongoing application of The Radiance Technique® supports a natural and radiant balancing, and a deeper relaxation of the entire physical-emotional-mental dynamic*

*from <u>within</u> to promote a reduction of stress. Expand to
twice daily sessions and add to your day several radiant
"breaks" to apply The Radiance Technique® while in the
working environment. Explore especially all of the Head
Positions whenever possible throughout the day, combined
with Front Positions #1 and/or #3.*[3]

Without a daily method for releasing stress and restoring
vital energy, most caregivers face the development of their
own health problems.

Care for the Caregiver

I often ask my caregiver clients if they have eaten that day. The
usual response is 'I grabbed a coffee' or 'There was no time.' I
try to get them to be partners in their care. Yes, maybe relaxing with a session of TRT® can help the headache they have,
but it could be caused by not eating, and so I encourage them
to do so. TRT® does not replace nutrition or sleep. A big myth
many women tell themselves is, "If I'm resting I must be lazy."
As noted earlier in the chapter, the additional responsibilities of work, family and household tasks, contribute to sleep
deprivation. Especially near the end and dying stages of their
loved one, there is practically no sleep at all for the caregiver.
Here we find another good reason to attend TRT® sessions.

TRT® is a replenishing energy support. Many clients are
completely exhausted and naturally fall asleep during a session. It is often in these quiet moments that many are able to
express how they are really feeling. Caregivers find it helpful
to connect to a support group, to meet with others, share and
know that they are not alone. A variety of support groups at
the Wellness Centre become invaluable to many and a lifeline
to get back to themselves.

The sessions of TRT® are nourishing and nurturing for
the caregiver, and for some, it gets them to begin to nourish
themselves. The time provides a sanctuary from their daily

demands. At the beginning of each session, they are told, "This is a time for you to relax, there is nowhere else you need to be, nothing else you need to do, just be here now." Sometimes, the support is just what they needed to get through the day. One caregiver summed up his experiences of TRT®in three words, "*Rested, relaxed and renewed.*"

Overall, caregivers have found relief of anxiety, pain relief, improved sleep patterns, increased awareness of stress, increased ability to nurture themselves, increased sense of well-being, release of tension, relaxation and a sense of peace. These all contribute to a higher quality of life that caregivers discover. Mary, whose sister was diagnosed with metastatic breast cancer, summed up her sessions in one remark: "It's been a *life-giving* experience."

"In Sickness and in Health..."

Barbara Bondy was referred to me in January 1997 from a social worker for emotional stress in dealing with her husband's diagnosis of lung cancer. Barbara found her sessions supportive, and they enabled her to get in touch with herself, especially in releasing her emotions. She found it getting harder to cope with her energy level so low. She felt the only time she rested was during her hour and an half session with me. Her energy level, like that of most caregivers, was very low, but she always kept on going, no matter what. Barb's caregiving journey with her husband was both challenging and transforming:

"We were high school sweethearts, first loves, only loves! We ran a business together and enjoyed raising four beautiful children. We were blessed with almost 24 years of a beautiful married life when we got the news: Ron had lung cancer. He was only forty-three! He was never sick a day in his life before this.

"'The denial. The anger. The 'life isn't fair, why doesn't God take all the rotten people in this world instead' syndrome began to set in. He survived a right lobectomy in London. I never left his side. We were together in health and we were going to beat this thing, too. Together, we were invincible. He was so strong. He wanted to live with his whole being.

"Six months later, the cancer metastasized to his left lung and through his bloodstream. The doctor said he could survive as little as two weeks and as long as one year. 'Every day after that is a gift,' the oncologist said. After five months of unsuccessful experimental chemotherapy with horrific results, we had to sell the business, our life.

"Every day was a struggle. His pain was unbearable, with bouts of vomiting blood for five hours at a time. We finally got in contact with Hospice. The case manager explained the services they had to offer. I was thoroughly intrigued with The Radiance Technique®. I was also very scared. Having been raised Catholic, I walked through most of my life with blinders on. What if this was hocus-pocus?

"Ron and I each had four sessions. Our lives took on a new direction. We found hope.

"From the very first session, I finally got in contact with my real emotions. From that moment on, I finally let myself feel and realize that yes, Ron was dying, and I had to help him die, and we had to live each day to the fullest and do and say everything to everyone. Ron and I were completely honest with each other throughout our lives, but illness opened a completely new world to his family. Each Radiant Touch® session brought all my emotions directly to the surface, and I felt every one of them intensely. My sessions were like a mini-dream.

"Ron looked forward to his ongoing sessions with Christine. She came to our house right up to the end. The sessions gave him hope and peace and even made his pain tolerable. He felt that he was not good enough to go to heaven. He thought that we would have to pray hard for him until he was good enough to get into heaven. How ridiculous! How incredible! Christine, through TRT®, calmed this fear. She made him

feel loved and deserving, and showed him that death is just a transition. His sick body was dying to rest but his vibrant soul would live on forever. She encouraged Ron to call our parish priest to come and talk to him.

"I watched Ron rot before my eyes, especially when the cancer spread to the bone, the kidneys, the brain and the heart. He suffered intensely, and we would have both gone insane without the loving support of family, friends and the Radiant Touch®. I took The First Degree Official Program of The Radiance Technique®, Authentic Reiki® on May 25, 1997, and it helped me to sleep at night. I used it on Ron, and it calmed us both down.

"Every day and every night, I used this wonderful healing, calming energy to accept the things I cannot change and go on and love the experience of the blessings of each day. I would never have chosen this walk in a million years, but there are people that I have been privileged to know and love that I would have had no need for had I chosen another path. The Radiance Technique® gives me a new perspective on life every time. The sun shines brighter, the grass grows greener, the breeze smiles warmer, the flowers smell more beautiful, and the birds fly more gracefully. Life is precious! The positive outlook — that even when in the bowels of despair the glint of sunshine, the tiny mustard seed of faith and hope grows; the love flourishes and the warm, caring depth of love and compassion found in all that Radiant energy sustains us and brings it all into the proper perspective.

"The pain of losing Ron was no greater than the joy of knowing and loving him. The Radiance Technique® gave me a positive attitude throughout the funeral, which was a beautiful celebration of his life. Ron illuminated love and generosity throughout his life. I chose to have his funeral mirror this. I wore white all three days, and the eulogy was funny, highlighting his wonderful sense of humour. We sang his favourite song in church, *Lord, It's Hard To Be Humble When You're*

Perfect In Every Way by Mac Davis. We let go two hundred white balloons depicting how very fragile life is, yet also how very strong and forever rising to greater heights. It also symbolized the resurrection. God said, *This is my beloved son of whom I am very proud.* I said, *This is my beloved husband of whom I am very proud.*

"The Radiance Technique® carried me and gave my children and me the courage, the stamina and the frame of mind to be a tribute to Ron's life. It also gave me the balance, the stress release, the willingness to go on and search once again for the joy in life."

Closer to Home

I remember the tireless commitment of a very special caregiver, Tina, my mom, when I was diagnosed with cancer. Both of my parents were amazing caregivers. My illness changed them and changed our relationship with each other. I remember sitting at the kitchen table years later and asking my mom how she felt at that time. She answered, "I just knew you would get better, and I was going to do everything in my power to help you." She later gave the same special caring and love to her father and mother who died five months apart. Now my mom's loving hands comfort others through her care. Even with TRT®, she serves as a role model for me:

"Having been a personal support worker for the past ten years, I provide all kinds of support to ill people in their home. Some of my duties consist of bathing clients, dressing and grooming, assisting with exercising and preparing meals. I don't think about it, but during my time in their home, I know that I am connecting with others in a unique way with my Radiant hands.

"I do hands-on while bathing a client's body or washing the hair, then I gently massage their back, arms and legs with lotion. Some clients have commented that my hands are warm and comforting; others say they feel soft and gentle. Each one I meet always receives some Radiant light and Cosmic Symbols.

"I've had several clients over the years that no one seems to be able to provide care to for one reason or another. The agency would label them as 'very difficult clients,' and I would get the call to go and see what I could do. It was amazing how they responded to me, and sometimes I'd even get a smile out of them.

"I believe my awareness has grown to be able to adjust myself, be flexible to each environment, to know what to do, put clients' needs first, not what is easier or faster. This is not something they train you for. My constant support has been my hands-on.

"My favourite position is the heart centre, Front Position #1. Since taking TRT®, I connect to my body and myself more. Given my non-traditional hours, I can be with a client at 6 a.m., have clients throughout the day and end my evening with another client at 9 p.m. In between, I rest with hands-on to rejuvenate myself in order to be able to give my one hundred percent to my clients."

Tina's use of Radiant Touch® shows the versatility of this technique. Every moment she is in contact with a client, she is generating Radiant energy through her touch. She also uses techniques that she studied in The Second Degree to support others at a distance.

Supporting from a Distance

Time and distance can be obstacles with some techniques when supporting a friend or family member who lives far away, but not with The Radiance Technique®. Wherever you are, once you have studied to The Second Degree Official Program of The Radiance Technique®, Authentic Reiki®, a whole new way of connecting and supporting others is open to you.

In The Second Degree training, an instructor teaches specific methods to direct transcendental energy to someone at a distance, whether across the room, across the city or on the other side of the world. This advanced level greatly expands the TRT®practitioner's capacity to give and share Radiant energy with no limitations. The student learns how to bring Radiant energy to any situation — past, present or future. In situations where hands-on cannot be easily applied, these advanced methods enable the practitioner to support a person by simply sitting by the bedside or across the room.

Mother Supports Daughter

Bonnie Browne and her husband have experienced an enormous amount of stress with their daughter's medical challenges; her body continuously produced benign tumours on her spine.

"My daughter suffers from a painful and debilitating disease for which medical science offers few answers. I was seeking alternative methods to help her with pain control when I was fortunate enough to discover The Radiance Technique®, which was being offered through the Hospice. My daughter received a few sessions, and she decided that it was helpful to her. I was thrilled to discover that I could learn TRT®and that a course was starting almost immediately.

"We don't always do a full hands-on together, but we often sit together in the evening, and I place my hand on the painful part of her back, and she finds this very soothing. During this time, I always direct energy to her as well.

"I find that I usually do TRT®on myself. While I am rarely able to complete a full hour session each day, I find that I can usually manage to have at least a twenty-minute session each morning on the four Head Positions. During this time, I often direct energy to someone whom I feel may particularly need it. I also often use the four Front Positions while I am sitting in meetings, church, etc. When practiced to some extent daily, it seems that regardless of life's stresses and strains, there seems to be a nucleus of calm within my centre.

"Last year, my daughter had two major surgeries — the first one scheduled for at least eight hours, the second one scheduled for ten hours. As soon as my husband and I settled into the waiting room, I placed my hands on my body in the general area of where I thought the surgery site was to be on Front Positions #3 and #4 and directed energy to her.

"The first surgery took just four hours, and the second about six hours, and she made an uncomplicated recovery from both. Coincidence?"

Spiritual Connection

Carole Tomajko volunteers with Hospice in *Kid's Can Cope*, a therapeutic support program that assists parents and their children connected to issues of illness. Carole, an engineer, just recently began her university studies in Pastoral Ministry.

"The richness of my experience with The Radiance Technique® began in earnest once I had received The Second Degree. The ability to use Cosmic Symbols and direct energy profoundly changed my understanding of this gift.

"The Cosmic Symbols [of TRT®] soon became an important part of my daily prayer life. My simple morning ritual begins with the lighting of candles, the reading of biblical excerpts with accompanying meditations, and the reading of additional meditation passages from famous and unknown sages of other spiritual belief systems. I follow this with silent prayer, in which I invite the Divine Mystery to speak to me.

"Once I had been taught the Cosmic Symbols, they were a beautiful addition to this sacred ritual. Following the lighting of my candles, I slowly circle my meditation room, and I outwardly pattern the Cosmic Symbols. I keep a basket of names near the candles which include individuals I direct energy to. I address their well-being through both TRT® and prayer. I repeat the Cosmic Symbols once I have completed my meditations and prayers.

"I also find myself directing the cosmic spiral to people during the day when I see they need a bit of energy. This includes stressed-out strangers, rude drivers and those who appear upset.

"Another unique opportunity with which I have been presented is my volunteer work with *Kids Can Cope*. I help with groups of ten or more and have the opportunity to quietly direct to all. With sufficient time, I can give entire sessions. With limited time, I can at the very least place my attention on the individual and radiantly connect them to love and light. I believe that a little bit of Radiant light can go a long way.

"The Radiance Technique® offers us the opportunity to offer light and love to others in any and all circumstances, regardless of the physical limitations of this plane of existence. I feel so fortunate to be cognizant of this powerful force."

A Lifetime Companion

Lois Comartin had been a volunteer with Hospice for 30 years, assisting and helping others on their journey when unexpectedly, she faced being on the other side. After a lifetime of marriage and companionship, she never thought that this experience would happen to her, and then her husband Don was diagnosed suddenly with lung cancer and brain metastasis. During her volunteering she had recommended TRT® to others for support, but it was not until she became a caregiver to her husband that she really knew what she was recommending.

Lois writes, "Now my family at Hospice offered me sessions of this wonderful technique, and this gift continued all through Don's illness and even after his death. The sessions would pick me up, dust me off and send me back to the many tasks at hand... and there are many when you care for a loved one, and all my family and friends too. It was an overwhelming time in my life. I received this 're-' experience once a week for four months. I call it this because it restores, refreshes, revitalizes, rebalances and relieves my pain, my stress and my tension among other things. I am sure that I would not be so mentally, physically and spiritually well were it not for this truly tender care given me.

"I was later offered a specialized training in TRT® through Hospice for volunteers. I jumped in the air and said 'of course' to the technique that saved my life. If I could do for others what they had done for me, that would be an honour.

"As a Hospice volunteer, my true love was always doing roster visitation with patients at the hospital with our oncology nurse June. Now, in the autumn of my life, having received so many gifts from the universe, I feel honoured to return gifts to those with whom I come in contact. Using my training in The Second Degree, I direct before I leave home to all I will encounter that day from the parking lot attendant to the security guard who waves 'so long' at the end of my day. Often throughout the day, there is only time for the spirituality with me to salute the spirit within others... but that's okay. As to the hands inside of my Hospice smock pocket, they are laid lovingly on those with whom I share my day.

"I consider this a great honour and a very humbling experience to be an instrument by which the Radiant energy can begin to comfort. Clients are almost filled with joy upon completion of a session and anxious to receive again. I feel that my spirituality somehow salutes the client's spirit, and for that hour we are as one, we are whole, we are a unit. At the same time, I, too, receive much peace and tranquility within.

It's a win-win situation if there ever was one!

"I now care for my hands in a much different manner. I no longer consider them 'my' hands; they are instruments for good and comfort. TRT® is a necessary support in my life, and the positive affect it produces on my whole body is truly amazing. Everything seems to return to perfect sync — body, mind, emotions and spirit once again join forces to meet the challenges and struggles of this life.

"In addition to my volunteer service, I work at a local funeral home as a hostess/greeter, and I often stand chatting with family and friends who are grieving. I am always giving mini-sessions (five to ten minutes) on people as we chat, and I see a calm about them afterwards as they move about. Have you ever heard the expression, 'They never knew what hit them?'. Well, I smile as I think, 'They never knew what calmed them!'

"One evening, a family member had flown in under terrible weather conditions and was filled with grief already. He was overcome with emotions at the sight of his dead brother and the sadness of his widow and children. With all of this emotional stress, being an epileptic, he was in danger of having a seizure. He was taken to one of our quiet rooms, and my boss requested TRT® be done. He was soon calmed enough to tell me all about his life and family back home. His anxiety and fears were decreasing as he drew energy from within himself, enough to continue through the next few days filled with experiences of love, tears, and laughter.

"Another gift The Second Degree gives me is the ability to direct to my loved ones, whether near or far, be it past, present or future.

"Awesome, totally awesome tools these Radiant hands of ours! All of this keeps me alert, aware and awake to the possibilities within me, allowing me to serve others better. The Radiance Technique® will carry me for as long as I am able to place my Radiant hands gently on my heart. I hope to be a giver for many years, to assist those who are in need of comfort."

Through Lois's journey with her husband, she realised the importance of caring for herself and accepting help. Caregiving takes a lot of energy. I remember how Lois was feeling; it was directly related to the health and stability of her husband. Her weekly sessions gave her balance, and, as she wrote, increased her ability to cope. We continued her sessions after Don's death; in fact, I saw her the day after. She was very fragile and felt her sessions assisted her in accepting her husband's death on a deeper level within her.

Expanding and Nurturing Self Awareness

Nancy Lauzon is a wife, mother, professional caregiver and teacher of students with visual impairment. TRT® helped deepen her marriage, enhance her caregiving and connect her to the silence within.

"Words seem so inadequate in describing what The Radiance Technique® has meant in my life these past four years," she says.

"Since my husband, Frank, completed The First Degree Official Program of The Radiance Technique®, Authentic Reiki®, our marriage of 31 years has taken on new meaning. Words say nothing about what the experience is. TRT® has become an integral part of our relationship and another method of communication on a deeper dimension of our being. Every day, we create time for hands-on, and even when we are sitting outside by our pool, we touch feet, elbows — our connection is magnified. I tried to think of the things that changed my life profoundly, like childbirth. TRT® has definitely profoundly changed my life in that I relate to my world around me differently.

"When children in my class have surgeries, I direct to them. As a professional caregiver, I use TRT® and its applications every day in all situations, environments both work, community and home, like a pebble dropped in water and ripples out and out. So many challenges that seem like insurmountable problems are resolved in ways that I could never imagine. Some difficulties take only a short time to work through, while others take much longer to reach a solution that is for the person's highest good. I am still learning every day the value of TRT®, but I know it is a part of my life that I will always cherish.

"Another observation in my own personal growth is how much more comfortable I am with silence in my daily life. I was never very comfortable with it and have always perceived myself to be quite articulate in talking about a variety of topics. Through the daily incorporation of TRT®, I am becoming quieter on both the outer and inner as I assume more the role of observer. I am witnessing and much more aware of the dynamic shifts that are occurring as TRT® transforms individuals and situations every day.

"The exciting discovery of experiencing such positive daily energy has reaffirmed my faith and increased my daily prayer. When I celebrated a birthday recently, I was keenly aware of how very different my life is now compared to before I encountered TRT®. I live my life choosing TRT® each day as an integral part of my existence. I feel that The Radiance Technique® is a means of bringing goodness to the world and inner peace to those in it."

Integrating TRT® in Daily Life

Joe Kornowski has now studied to The Third Degree - 3A. His unfolding journey of TRT® supports his wife, his service to others and his daily life.

"Professionally, I was trained as a lawyer and have practiced law, served as a bar association executive, and helped develop law-related technology products. In my inner life, I have experienced the mystery and adventure of a journey towards the unknown for many years. My own journey has brought knowledge and insights from practices of Christian mysticism, Zen meditation, Tai Chi, Native American medicine and, more recently, The Radiance Technique®.

"One of the more profound insights and resulting changes that The Radiance Technique® has provided me is a deeper-but-'lighter' understanding of service to others. Before studying TRT®, I mostly equated service with personal sacrifice, a kind of giving up of my own time, priorities, and interests to a greater or lesser extent, in order to help another. The other's gain, I believed, was necessarily at my expense on one or more levels. In fact, it was precisely this self-sacrifice element that I thought made service so honourable, admirable and laudable, along with the self-satisfaction of knowing I had helped a fellow human being.

"Since studying TRT®, however, I have come to know service not as self-sacrifice but rather as *self-expression and self-expansion.* Instead of a sacrifice of my own time, priorities and interests, I now see such service more clearly as an alignment of them in a way that supports others while deepening and expanding myself. I feel the responsibility to help bring Light where it appears to be needed. And I see that in sharing my own flame to spread Light to others, I do not lose anything. In fact, it actually feels as if my own Light burns a little more brightly when I am sharing it with another, whether I know that person or not, and whether they know I am doing so or not. Maybe it is simply the growing awareness that my Light, when I share it, becomes our Light.

"It is this new experience and resulting understanding since studying The Second Degree that has compelled me to do several directing sessions daily — some one-to-one, as well as collectively to those I want to support on an on-going basis. Somehow, through TRT®, my expanding need and desire to serve has changed from 'going out of my way' to simply 'my way.' Whether during the day from my office or at home in the evening or on weekends, I find it is an excellent way to stay connected and focused on my own awakening journey.

"My more immediate and personal service, however, is with my wife, who has suffered from a chronic lung disease for the past several years, as well as bursitis in her shoulder, and panic/anxiety disorder, which often makes it difficult for her to leave the house. Consequently, I do most of the grocery shopping and other errands for us.

"Since studying TRT®, I have been able to support her in various ways, including sharing a hands-on session. She generally prefers hands-on her shoulder, knees, back, ribs, or feet. She has commented that, even if she has me place my hands on one particular area of her body, she always notices significant improvement, such as pain relief, in other areas that may also be bothering her. With my Second Degree expansion, I have begun simultaneously to direct to other areas while doing hands-on in a specific area.

"At other times, when her breathing seems laboured or she otherwise seems uncomfortable or in pain but prefers me not to do hands-on, I will begin directing to her and patterning the cosmic symbols internally while sitting next to her watching television. Additionally, I will pattern the Cosmic Symbols in the bedroom before she comes to bed, focusing particularly on her side of the bed and her pillow, as well as her favourite place on the couch.

"Typically, I make us both dinner, or else bring it in. In either case, I will pattern Cosmic Symbols over the food or do hands-on before serving it. Supporting her in these ways not only is part of my caring for her, but it has deepened our connection and provided me new strength and insight in dealing with the challenges of her chronic disease.

"In addition to its impact on my caring for my wife and serving others, TRT® has brought about a change in my understanding of death. The first time that I reached out through a directing session to someone who had made her transition was with an aunt, as part of an exercise in my Second Degree class. I saw directly, and for the first time as a personal experience, the *continuum of human existence*. What struck me most was that there was no real break in that existence, certainly no true "end" in the way that I had thought of death as bringing a final termination to human existence. I saw that the form of that existence was certainly different from a living being; it seemed almost that I was connecting to the pure essence of the person I had known as my aunt, free of the personality traits and idiosyncrasies that I had associated with her in this world. I realized that I had connected with her at a level other than as two worldly personalities who were related by blood.

"On a different level, she still exists. She remains accessible and available for me to connect with. That realization has surfaced myriad possibilities for my continued expansion and awakening — and service — through connection with those who were personally important to me when they were living, as well as with enlightened beings who I never knew personally and who are no longer physically in this world but are nevertheless accessible and available to me.

"In this regard, TRT® and most recently The Second Degree expansion already have made a profound difference in how I go about my daily life in a more integrated, healing and whole way — for myself, for my wife and for others. Not merely a change in my actions or behaviour, my use of TRT® seems to be facilitating a change in my very being."

Coordinating Service with TRT®

One of the first voices clients will hear at the other end of the phone at Hospice is Service Coordinator, Linda Sabatini. She has been with Hospice for over 20 years and provides program coordination in the Wellness Centre as well as support to the clinical team. Linda has supported many patients and their families over the years and always takes time to listen. "With gratitude and appreciation I was given the gift of learning The Radiance Technique®. This was a gift of honouring self-worth. Learning TRT®was an extension of my belief of self-healing, self-awareness and spiritual awakening. I have strengthened my want for inner balance, true self-connection, authenticity and empowerment.

"Consciously and unconsciously I integrate a blending of the hand positions in both my professional and personal well-being. I feel a greater sense of peace and harmony with those around me and within myself.

"As Service Coordinator I respond to and address the needs of patients and their families accessing our services. I work with a team of health care professionals in developing a plan of care to support, educate and empower. We ensure their quality of care.

"I am consciously aware from the moment I engage with a patient either by phone or in person, that I am fully connected to them on all levels. While on the phone, I can speak with a calming, supportive and sympathetic voice by holding my hand on my heart centre.

"When I meet patients and families, whether I shake or hold their hand, the Radiant energy is flowing. In sitting with them, I may have my hands open facing them or on Front Position #1 as I flow energy, allowing and giving permission for them to share freely within confidence.

"Both as giver and receiver of The Radiance Technique®, I experience a heightened awareness of the energy around me. It brings balance and weaving wholeness to my mental, physical, emotional and spiritual well-being.

"I have used Radiant Touch®with my father who is living with cancer. It is with thankfulness and privilege that I can support him in affirming his wish and want for a better quality of life and well-being. This has given me the wisdom to live with courage, strength and love as I go through this sacred journey with him. I live with the knowledge and true blessings of a father/daughter connection."

Linda's sharing is echoed by the words of Christine Longacker in her book, *Facing Death and Finding Hope*, who writes, "But we, the caregivers, are not the only givers. Sooner or later, all who work with dying people know they are receiving more than they are giving as they meet endurance, courage, and often humour. We need to say so, recognizing too the common conviction that there is an enabling grace coming from beyond us both."[4]

Life's Unfolding Process

Katherine Lenel writes of TRT®'s contribution with her father before, during and after his transition.

"The Radiance Technique® is a profound support for the 'cared for' and for the caregiver," she observes. "Especially in the circumstances of relating to a parent who is in the process of dying, many kinds of awareness may be experienced, and deep experiences of healing are possible. I share the following about my caregiving role with my father using TRT®.

"My father and I share a deep bond of love and in struggle over very different views of life and its meaning. Five years ago, he suffered a series of heart attacks and seemed very close to death. I was unable to be with him physically, and I experienced periods of time in which I was very frightened about his impending transition. I was afraid he would die afraid, and I found this thought intolerable. I wanted to spare him unhappiness. At this time, I began a regular practice of directing energy to him every evening.

"In relation to this practice, I had a series of realizations about our relationship that have freed me ever since. I realized that he had his own life to live. As much as I had suffered from his inability to recognize my right to live my life my own way, he suffered from my refusal to allow him, in my mind, to make his choices in responding to his life. I knew I could not 'spare' him the consequences of his thoughts and actions anymore than he could 'spare' me mine. I could love absolutely from my heart, and, in wholeness, I could accept him exactly the way he really was. TRT®was the tool that allowed me to see and to release the dense patterns of my interaction with my father.

Private letter to the author, 1998: "In 1998, at the age of 91, my father has been placed in a nursing home for patients with dementia. His very fine mind often wanders, and my mother is no longer able to care for him. To see him losing the powers of his mind and body, which were so much his during most of life, is sad for me. It pulls at my emotional heart. Yet, I can still direct energy to him and know him for what he is, at least in this cycle on earth: loving, irascible, clever, impatient, full of integrity, obdurate, demanding and conscientious — a being of great contrasts, unrepeatable. And he can be held in the warmth of universal love as he lives out the full cycle of his time on earth.

Private letter to the author, 2003: "March, [2003] my father made his transition, The Radiance Technique®is helping with every aspect of this event. My mother, and two of my sisters and I were with my father for most of two days as he lay dying. I was able to use physical hands-on with him for many hours during those days, and although he was not able to speak, or, as far as I could tell, to see clearly during that time, he definitely moved toward me and my hands, and became calmer as I touched him with radiant hands. I used the Cosmic Symbols that I knew from advanced levels of study of The Radiance Technique®when I sat with my father, and also during the times my sisters and mother and I spent together at meals.

"None of us slept well during this time, and the gentle, sustaining energy of TRT® is what supported us in a positive frame of mind. On the first afternoon, when I arrived, my father's room at the assisted-living facility was filled with family members and hospice care workers, yet when I began to use TRT® with my dad, and when he became more and more peaceful, all of the other people gradually filed out of the room and left me to continue to share TRT® with him. Later, a nurse from the facility stopped by to administer morphine to my father, and spoke with me as if I were a hospice nurse. I told him that I was Fritz's daughter, *i.e.,* a family member, and he was very surprised. He said he had heard from the hospice workers and others on the nursing staff that I was a special hospice nurse from Florida who was really helping Fritz to rest! My father made his transition a day and a half later.

"The weeks since his transition have been full of opportunities for emotional and spiritual growth. I was mentally aware before his death, that the passing of a parent can prompt significant changes in one's experience of one's own life — yet my experience has been quite different from what I might have imagined. My awareness of the 'background noise' in my mind during much of my day has heightened, and I have felt that I am only now seeing my 'little' self and my mental and emotional habits with clarity. I use The Radiance Technique® many times a day — both the hands-on technique and the Cosmic Symbols and attunement processes — to allow myself to centre and focus on what is actually happening inside me. Often, the ability to see how I am really feeling and thinking in a situation is enough to allow me to drop painful habits that I have practiced since my childhood. Sometimes I am aware of thoughts and attitudes that are powerfully negative due to long cultivation. The relaxation and feeling of 'interior space' which so often comes when I use TRT®, allows me to stay steady with fears, resentment and other unpleasant emotions and *'Trust in my life's unfolding process'*, a phrase which I

learned through a very early issue of *The Radiance Technique*®
Journal. In *The Expanded Reference Manual of The Radiance
Technique*®, *Authentic Reiki*®, there is an entry for the term
'Opportunity.' The entry concludes,

> *The Radiance Technique*®, *whenever it is used by you, gives
> an opportunity for natural growth, for expansion and trans-
> formation according to your needs, for increasing your
> caring, loving and nurturing qualities and for supporting
> <u>all</u> aspects and polarities of your cycles in Real Light.*[5]

"This describes my experience of using The Radiance
Technique® since my father's death. I am learning self care,
Acceptance and a great deal about the privilege we are given
to live the life of a human being on the planet Earth.

"It is clear to me, especially after reading what I have written about these experiences, that The Radiance Technique®
has facilitated, and is facilitating, a deep process of discovery
about illusion and true identity. What a wonder and privilege
it is to reach out with TRT® to another and in the process to
discover oneself!"

Dr. Barbara Ray has given specific and practical sugges-
tions for TRT® Hands-on positions throughout *The Expanded
Reference Manual of The Radiance Technique*®, *Authentic
Reiki*®. Some of these include:

Relaxation and Calming:

A whole session when possible, plus extra time in Head
Positions #2 and #3 and Front Positions #1 and #3.

Balancing:

A whole session, plus extra time with one hand at Head
Position #3 and one at Front Position #3.

Physical Pain:

Emphasis on Head Positions #2 and #3 and Front Positions #1, #2, #3.

Mental Confusion:
Head Positions #1, #2, and #3 and Front Position #3.

Fatigue:
A whole session, plus extra time on Head Positions #1, #2, and #3

Supporting others along the way, as Katherine and others shared, can be an opportunity for healing and discovery. However, we are only as good as what we do to care for ourselves. I offer the following suggestions to support you as a caregiver:

Caring Suggestions for Caregivers:
Getting the Help You Need
In addition to your restoring and renewing sessions of The Radiance Technique®, consider the following:

- Accept support. You do not have to do it alone.
- Ask for help from neighbours, friends, relatives and volunteer organizations. Let others provide support, others who have walked the path before you. Let people know what you need. Be specific, such as: *I need someone to pick up the kids on Monday and Wednesday nights,* or *I need someone to prepare lunch five days a week.*
- If you are working, discuss options with your employer to minimize stress and have more flexibility. Many companies have Employee Assistance Programs that can give you support.
- It is very helpful to talk to someone outside your family and friends. Counselling can help make the journey smoother and allows you to freely express yourself without being judged. Social Workers can also guide you in finding the right resources or medical personnel

you need. They are a part of services provided by hospices and cancer centres.

- Join a caregiver support group.
- Receive spiritual nourishment from whatever your beliefs and religious practices are. Prayer, healing words, and books of encouragement will support you.
- Play or listen to a variety of music and tap into music's healing abilities. Check out the back of the book for recommended Music Resources.
- Balance your life with humour. Laughing and looking at the lighter side of life is healing.
- Appreciate the little every day experiences and miracles.
- To help maintain optimum energy at this time, remember the big three: R.E.D.

Rest

- Get adequate sleep. If you don't sleep, the whole mind-body suffers. It's best to be in bed by 10 p.m. Ask friends or volunteers to sit with your loved one while you get some sleep.

Exercise

- Exercise between your care times. Every little bit helps. Try walking, biking, swimming, yoga or tai chi. Stretching and moving your body decreases stress and increases energy.

Diet

- The saying 'you are what you eat' applies. Eat freshly prepared organic foods. Avoid canned foods, frozen foods, leftovers, and cooking with microwaves.
- Have your largest meal of the day at noon with a lighter meal at dinner. If you eat meat, have it at noon for optimum digestion.
- Eat in a relaxed atmosphere and don't rush.

Drink

- Drink water throughout the day at a level comfortable for you. You can have a flask of warm water to sip on throughout the day. According to Ayurvedic medicine, taking two sips of warm water every half hour cleanses the digestive track which improves your digestion and assimilation of food.

- Avoid caffeine altogether or take in small amounts. Drinks with caffeine stimulate the nervous system and give a false sense of energy to your body. This causes you to draw upon energy you do not have, disrupting your natural ability to know when you need to rest.

- Spice Water: A general tea taught to me by Dr. Paul Dugliss, M.D., has many benefits for improving digestion and overall well-being:

  - Boil 1½ quarts of water and place in thermos flask. Add the following spices: ½ teaspoon coriander(seeds), 1tsp. fennel seeds and ¼ tsp. cumin seeds. Leave in flask and drink throughout the day. Discard at 6 pm and prepare fresh the next morning.

- Fresh organic juices are a good way to get nutrients into your body.

- Avoid alcohol in evenings. It stimulates your system in the long run rather than calming your body and often increases depression.

And one last suggestion try:

- Daily Self-Massage.
  In Ayurvedic medicine, self-massage or *Abhyanga*, is an oil massage that has many benefits. It calms your nerves, improves mental alertness and promotes a better night's sleep. It is also a way to nurture yourself. This is an easy massage that anyone can do, as there are really only two main movements:

- Circular motions over round areas like your head, stomach and joints
- Straight up-and-down strokes over your limbs — arms and legs

Follow these simple steps:

- Warm up your oil by placing your bottle in a cup of hot water. It is best to pour the amount you need in a plastic flip-top bottle, that way you are not heating up your large bottle every day. Suggestion: use organic safflower oil purchased from a reputable source.
- Apply the oil while standing in the bathtub or shower area.
- Place warmed oil in your hands and begin by massaging your scalp, face, ears and neck. Begin at the top and work your way down. Be generous with the oil.
- Apply oil to your entire chest and stomach as well as your back (as much as you can) and then do your arms, hips, thighs and legs stroking up and down and then circular movements on the joints. Remember to massage your feet and hands.
- Let the oil stay on your body for at least ten minutes, then take a warm shower, or you may towel it off. It is recommended to perform this massage first thing in the morning. Refrain from applying during your menstrual cycle.

For additional suggestions, seek the support of a qualified Natural Health Physician or Health Educator who will guide you in restoring balance according to your body type.

¹ Article: "Why Having a National Home Care Program is a Women's Issue", by Jean Ann Lowry, The Network, Spring/Summer 2002 Volume 5, number 2/3 p. 6. Canadian Women's Health Network.

² Article: "A Woman's Guide to Health Care Debates" by Pat Armstrong, *The Network*, Spring/Summer 2002, Volume 5, number 2/3, p. 13. Canadian Women's Health Network.

³ Ray, *The Expanded Reference Manual of The Radiance Technique*®, *Authentic Reiki*®, p. 17.

⁴ Longacker, Christine, *Facing Death and Finding Hope*, (New York, NY: Doubleday 1997), p. 228.

5 Ray, *The Expanded Reference Manual of The Radiance Technique*®, *Authentic Reiki*®, p. 79.

Be a lamp, or a lifeboat, or a ladder.
Help someone's soul heal.
Walk out of your house like a shepherd.

~ Rumi
'Diwan-i Shams-i Tabriz-i'

Social Workers: Partners in Care

*It is my experience that
The Radiance Technique® moves us
into a place of possibility, which is the
deeper awareness and inner knowledge
spiritually of the truth of who we really are.
It assists with the movement into a
place of peace and tranquillity
because we can remember
our essence as Spiritual Beings
completing a physical life while
having mental and emotional
reactions as we face our
various challenges.*

~ *Jan Dennis, Social Worker*

-5-

SOCIAL WORKERS IN THE HOSPICE FIELD are caring companions along the journey, providing a listening ear and psychosocial support to patients and their families. They are bridge builders by helping people access practical services and maneuveur in the health care system. They are sounding boards for thoughts, feelings and spiritual concerns to be expressed and explored. When social workers use The Radiance Technique®, their professional and personal lives are enhanced and their capacities for expanded supportive care are deepened. This chapter reveals the support of TRT® experienced by social workers in Windsor and abroad, both during and after work hours.

Remembering My Essence

Jan Dennis, M.S.W., C.S.W., was a Hospice Consultant in Windsor and studied to The Second Degree of TRT®. She provided care, innovative support programs and services for over 20 years. Jan wrote this sharing in 2004.

"I have been involved with The Radiance Technique® as a professional clinical social worker as I recommend that cancer patients and their family members receive this therapy. This evolved when I completed the training of The First Degree Official Program of The Radiance Technique®, Authentic Reiki®. However, the most significant experience came very recently when I needed to receive TRT® myself as a result of my younger and closest sister's diagnosis of melanoma.

"TRT® helped me to be able to remember the essence of

living this life. It helped me also to focus on my inner self and fed my spirit so that I could help my sister and at the same time function by continuing to meet my obligations professionally until the stress was alleviated.

"I believe that the first consideration in examining TRT® is that it is universal in nature. Beyond my own personal experience and 30 years of professional experience, The Radiance Technique® enjoys an acceptance across cultural, educational, social, spiritual, mental, emotional and physical boundaries, which for all other techniques produce limitations and constraints. I have for many years continued to hear from clients facing cancer how TRT® has significantly impacted and helped them during such a difficult and stressful time in their lives.

"It is my experience that The Radiance Technique® moves us into a place of possibility, which is the deeper awareness and inner knowledge spiritually of the truth of who we really are. It assists with the movement into a place of peace and tranquillity because we can remember our essence as Spiritual Beings completing a physical life while having mental and emotional reactions as we face our various challenges.

"The Radiance Technique® is a gift. It assists with the need to return to the place where our inner knowingness can help us to integrate as a physical, mental, emotional, social and spiritual being.

"With this integration comes the possibility of re-awakening the sense of awe, the experience of inner peace and the need to explore the mysteries of life."

Returning to My Centre

Maggie Johnson, B.S.W., R.S.W., integrates TRT® into the care plan for her clients and for herself. In the summer of 2002, Maggie received the news that she had breast cancer. "I knew immediately that my treatment would include conventional as well as complementary modalities. Throughout the nine months of my chemo and radiation, I had regular Radiant Touch® sessions in my home. I looked forward to these sessions as they always calmed, balanced and rejuvenated my body and spirit. As well, on the rare occasions that I would wake in the night with some fear or restlessness, a few minutes of hands-on soon put me back to sleep. Now two years post treatments, I am feeling wonderful and all of my tests point to the fact that my immune system is working well. I continue to include hands-on time as part of my day."

Maggie's background includes ten years as a social worker with Hospice in Windsor and another ten years as a patient care volunteer. She has been a member of the organization Woman Within International, Inc., and has facilitated many groups. She has a special interest in supporting others as they weave their way through the diagnosis, treatment and recovery processes. Maggie is now in private practice and offers innovative support programs for patients, especially for women with breast cancer.

"When I interview clients for the first time, there are several scenarios that suggest to me that a referral to Radiant Touch® is appropriate. When anxiety is at such a level that there is an inability to focus thoughts, extreme fear regarding diagnosis or treatment, difficulty sleeping or inability to think of anything other than the illness and possible death, I will refer right away. My experience is that the majority of those referred are soon demonstrating much less anxiety. I have also referred people who are depressed and cannot muster the energy to complete daily tasks. Often, they tell me after a few sessions that their energy level has increased.

"Another group I refer are those who are very self-aware, who know that something needs to change in their view of self or their world if they are to heal. They often report very important insights into themselves and their lives because of their Radiant Touch® sessions.

"I have had occasions when I went into homes to interview patients and found them unable to process much of what I was saying in terms of services. In that event, I will explain TRT® and offer to demonstrate by doing the Head Positions and Front Position #1. They not only calm considerably enough to hear about some other components of services, but they request more Radiant Touch® sessions.

"In my personal life, TRT® is one of a number of modalities I use to keep me grounded and connected to spirit. I frequently incorporate Head Positions #1 and #2 and Front Positions #1 to #4 into my yoga and meditation practices. In addition, when my work is stressful, I will close my office door and take a few minutes to do the Head Positions and find that this helps me refocus and brings me back to my centre."

TRT® Gives Needed Energy

Jean Whittal, B.S.W., C.D.C., Canadian Mental Health community support worker and cancer survivor reveals her personal expansion with TRT® and her experiences during her position as a Hospice social worker.

"In 1995, I became an employee as a case manager," she explains. "Part of my job was introducing the programs that Hospice offered. I wanted to experience as many of the programs as possible to help me explain the benefits of each one to clients.

"After experiencing TRT®, I wanted to learn how to become a practitioner. That year, I took The First Degree Official Program of The Radiance Technique®, Authentic Reiki®. It not only helped me to explain it to my clients but also became a part of my daily life. TRT® taught me how to relax and become aware of the true meaning of wholeness. My total body would relax; my mind slowed down, my focus was clear, and my senses attuned to my surroundings. A peaceful feeling was within me. My sense of colour and scent enhanced greatly. I learned to become more patient and accepting of others. Inside and out, I felt centred.

"I am a cancer survivor. At the age of 35, I received the diagnosis of bowel cancer. After a recurrence, I decided nothing in life was worth worrying over and became more relaxed and closer to nature. This was lost when I decided to go to university and become a social worker. My mother became ill, and with constant care-giving and a heavy workload from classes, I became Type A person again. TRT® brought me back to the reality of what I needed to do to stay well.

"Cancer of the bowel weakens your digestive system and can rob you of much-needed nutrients. I use Front Positions #3 and #4 most often to help the functioning of my bowels. TRT® helps with the digestion and constipation. I can eat almost every type of food and have gained weight.

"While counselling clients, giving myself TRT® enables me to focus better and look at situations more objectively and subjectively. Each client I work with requires different levels of energy; TRT gives the needed energy. Clients become aware of my serenity and calm state, which reduces their anxiety and stress. The free flow of energy transcends into peace and tranquillity, leading to a helpful and productive counselling session.

"I often give Radiant Touch® to those who live in the county and are too ill to make the trip into the city. Each situation is different. For those who are in the end stage of life, TRT® offers freedom from pain whether it is physical, emotional, spiritual or psychological, or death anxiety and loneliness. The following people have touched my life as I theirs using my radiant hands.

"Joan was end-stage heart disease when she was referred to me by the Victorian Order of Nurses. Joan was very weak, pale and in pain. I explained to Joan what I was going to do, and she was very receptive. I gave her the usual four Head Positions and gave extra time to Front Position #1 and Back

Position #1 for the heart centre. After the first session, Joan was looking less stressed, appeared to be calm and smiled. She stated that the pressure and pain in her chest was relieved.

"Joan was on experimental drugs that she thought were keeping her alive. The Ministry of Health would no longer endorse the drugs because of the severe side effects. Joan's doctor told her she would die soon. She had a warm and loving family, but as the end grew near, they spent less time with her. Joan knew they were not comfortable with death or seeing her suffer. It was lonely for her.

"As time passed, each TRT® session helped Joan with her emotional and physical pain. She became more forgiving of her family, and the pains in her chest grew weaker. After each session, she would talk about her past, present and preparation for death. As time went on, I continued with sessions and observed Joan was growing weaker. TRT® brought us closer. She knew I was comfortable with her and not afraid of death. She was dying, and I was living, both together but on different planes of energy. The transcending of the light energy given and received put us in an equal state as one. There was total trust and love.

"Joan was not afraid to die, but when we first began, she wanted to live longer. She stated TRT® helped her to accept her time was near, and she took care of all her affairs.

"The last time I gave Joan Radiant Touch®, it had been five months after her drugs were stopped, and she knew her time to die was approaching. She had a warm and loving smile and a radiant glow around her head. I stared at her in amazement, which broadened her smile. Was this cosmic awareness and total consciousness? Joan died that night. We both knew it that day and said our good-byes. I will never forget Joan or her angelic look.

"Another client I would like to share about is James. My first visit with James was not a productive one. He had had an argument with his adult children and was very angry. James was a man of few words and a private person. He had a tumour growing out of his back and could only sit and lie in one position. He really did not want me there and asked me to leave. I respected his wish but before I left, I asked him if I could come back. He knew I accepted his anger and was genuinely concerned for him. I briefly explained to him that I thought I had something that would help, The Radiance Technique®.

"I set up an appointment and gave him TRT®. Before we started, James told me that he did not have any feeling in his legs and feet. I gave him the usual twelve positions and then four added positions: the Front Positions #1 and #4 to support his anger, frustration and stress reduction. Then, I placed my hands on both his legs and feet.

"James was lying on his stomach while receiving TRT®, and he was reading his Bible. When I finished, James was astonished. He had experienced feeling in both his legs and feet. As he was reading his Bible, he found new meaning and clarity in the verses. As time passed, James's anger decreased, and he showed a sense of humour. James got some of his personality back and found new meaning in his experiences.

"Using hands-on helps replenish my energy, listen more effectively and be more aware of client's energy while working with their different levels of consciousness. Each morning, I use the cosmic symbols to direct energy to my coworkers and clients. It improves the relationships and opens up communication that is more effective. Creative ideas appear and help clients process their feelings and be in the here and now.

"I have also directed Radiant energy to friends and family. My brother recently became ill due to stress and long hours at work. I directed to him without his knowing. He informed me that he was coming home from work, eating his dinner and going directly to bed. He was sleeping well and getting rest he so desperately needed.

"In my own illness, there were several struggles with the physical, emotional, mental and spiritual pain. Recently, I came to accept the fact that I might die. It was only then my spirit came back, the physical pain decreased, and my consciousness awoke. I enjoyed every sight and sound, and I had no sense of time. Freedom from fear and anxiety left. My experiences affirmed for me that my soul is not my physical body.

"TRT® has given me a new level of understanding about how to be more aware of the universe, self and others, and a raised sense of consciousness. TRT®, used with social work, enhances the therapeutic relationship with trust, change and acceptance. Once you have learned, TRT® will remain with you permanently and will always bring inner peace. The Radiance Technique® is the road to self-actualization and the tool to help you get there while helping others achieve their own self-actualization whether living or dying."

The many ways that Radiant Touch® and other capacities of TRT® are applied at home and at work emphasize the science's versatility. "In her foreword to the book, *The Radiance Technique® on the Job*, Barbara Ray, Ph.D., expresses the support that TRT® has given to alumni who have applied it in their daily lives to promote the 'release of tension and stress, to expand job creativity and productivity, to renew and revitalize their energy levels all day in their work environments....'"[1]

TRT® Balances

Stephen Brennen, M.S.W., R.S.W., currently serves as Director of The Centre of Excellence at Hospice. He has supported patients and families for over 20 years and uses TRT® for self-help: "I continue to use my training in The Second Degree for personal growth and balance. It has assisted greatly in maintaining my energy flow as I interact with others in my role as a psychotherapist. I recommend it readily to clients, particularly those going through major life transitions. It has benefited many that are dealing with cancer, heart disease and HIV/AIDS by providing balance in their struggle with the life changes inherent with illness and even in death."

Couples Support

For Ruth Ann Wilhelm, M.S.W., R.S.W., personal growth and development have been integral to her life. In 1983, she began her involvement with Pathwork, an organization focused on personal transformation. Subsequently, she developed an interest in the mind-body-spirit connection and studied reflexology and The Radiance Technique®. She has supported many through her work over the years as a social worker and now is supporting her husband.

"When my husband was diagnosed with aggressive prostate cancer, I signed up to learn TRT® so that I could be helpful to him with the process of treatment and its side effects. Imagine my surprise; when I attended the first class, the teacher recommended it first for personal care and relaxation. Of course, it was a lesson that I needed to learn. It's like the instructions they provide on the airplane all the time. In the event of an emergency, fasten your own oxygen mask first and then go on to help others. And so that is what I have tried to do.

"TRT® has been essential for me each time, in the days after a new aspect of my husband's diagnosis or test results are given. When I feel the fear and terror building, I do a full session for myself in the moment. And when I cannot sleep at night, I do it to relax and usually fall back to sleep.

"Six months after first learning TRT®, I signed up to learn The Second Degree and immediately applied the expanded energy techniques to my life and husband's situation.

"For about a month, he had been struggling with his continence, the result of a radical prostatectomy. His continence had improved after surgery but several months later and, for no apparent reason, it deteriorated. After a month of three different medications, alone and in combination, there was no sustained improvement. Desperate because the bathroom was controlling our lives, he was in pain each time he went, and he was beginning radiation treatment, I used all that I had learned in The Second Degree. I held his medication and supplements and patterned cosmic symbols with them for about 15 minutes. Then I patterned cosmic symbols throughout the house, over the toilet, over his side of the bed, over the chairs he sat in and over the massage table. I spent about three hours patterning and doing hands-on myself. In addition, I shared a hands-on session with him, gave him a reflexology treatment, and directed TRT® to him. I also directed to the decisions he needed to make about his continence and medications. By the next day there was gradually increasing improvement. His continence is nowhere near pre-surgery but it is more manageable. And as he continues in radiation therapy, it is remarkable that he has the limited side effects that he does!

"Another way that TRT® has been helpful for me is with service to others. When someone shares about any health concern, I add the name and situation to my directing list and feel relieved that I can offer support in this way at a time in my life when I have less available energy for physical support. I take comfort in the fact that each time I direct Radiant energy I am including positive energy for my entire immediate and extended family and the range of their needs. When I feel distress about seeing dead animals on the side of the road, I do cosmic symbols to support their spirit. If I feel anxious in the car, when traveling, or about an impending encounter, I do the symbols, again to support the highest good.

"I believe that my life is much improved in living the current circumstances. TRT® has expanded my understanding of energy, of its timeless nature, and the energy component in every aspect of life and living."

Opening Heart for Healing

Joanne McGuire, B.S.W., a social worker at the Windsor Regional Cancer Centre, has been supporting people for many years, first as a Hospice volunteer and then as a staff member.

"I completed The First Degree Official Program of The Radiance Technique®, Authentic Reiki®, in March 2001. I have been using TRT® for my own self-care and to see how I may be able to apply it to the patients and family members I work with.

"Initially, I was a bit nervous to use TRT® on the patients because of time constraints and in explaining the technique. I decided not to worry too much about it and just trust that, in time, it would start to flow. What I did notice is that after taking TRT®, it was much clearer to me how I could speak about TRT® to patients and family members before making a referral to the Hospice Radiant Touch® program.

"Upon visiting one of my patients, whose wife I had recently made a referral for TRT®, I found him to be in distress and uncomfortable. I could sense that the end of his life was near and recognized some of the signs of death anxiety. This gentleman was unable to speak at this time, but you could tell from his facial expressions that he and his wife were in distress.

"I walked over to his bed, and I gently explained that I was going to do a relaxation technique in hopes that it would calm him. I explained to him what I was going to do with my hands and the various positions on his body that I would place them. I explained that I did not have to touch his body, so he had no need to be concerned about me possibly hurting him since he was in a very fragile condition.

"I placed my hands on Head Position #1, and I could feel a tremendous amount of heat. It was emanating from his body. At first, I thought it was because the weather was hot and humid. In hindsight, however, I think it was his life energy moving in his body, and I will explain this more later on. I asked his wife if she could put on some of his favorite music for comfort, and she obliged.

"As I continued with the positions, I experienced an

enormous amount of heat in the head and front upper chest positions. As I moved to the lower part of his body, I was aware of the lack of warmth/heat there. Not wanting to judge that anything was wrong, I continued to hold my hands over this part of his body and invited his wife to come over and sit with him and hold his hand. While doing TRT®, I realized that this man was dying and that his wife needed to be near him. I had spent a lot of time with these two courageous people and knew of the deep bond and love between them; it was important for her to be part of this.

"I could not help but feel that by doing Radiant Touch®, a peaceful environment was created not only for the patient but also for his wife and myself. It allowed me to centre and become peaceful and to focus on the wife. I also felt that it provided an opportunity to be with my patient in such a way that could provide an opportunity for transformation to occur even though I could not say what that was. It felt holy, peaceful and loving.

"The patient died about eight hours later. I have never forgotten this experience. It was the starting point for me to continue training in the field of energy and to broaden my capacity of being with people. It has also helped me from a spiritual perspective. I often use Front Position #1, the heart position, on others and myself. I believe that having an open heart benefits us in so many ways, and find I am drawn to this position as well as Front Position #3, the solar plexus position.

"At this point in time, I have also trained in Therapeutic Touch™. However, my TRT® experience has provided me with a foundation that supports my own spiritual, personal and professional development. I incorporate it into my work and use it for my own personal support as well. Death and dying is a sensitive area to work in at an emotional level, and I find having TRT® and other energy modalities available helps to support me from a wholistic perspective in balancing and to maintaining an open heart."

Radiant Support in Dying

Brigitte Strobel works as a social worker, has studied to
The Fourth Degree, and is an Authorized Instructor of The
Radiance Technique® in Berlin, Germany. Each day is an
opportunity to apply TRT® in her daily life and profession.

"Over a period of three weeks, I had the great privilege
of sharing Radiant Touch® with a man in his dying process,"
explains Brigitte. "He and his wife were both familiar with
TRT® in receiving hands-on sessions as well as having The
Second Degree. On my first visit, he was lying in bed. He was
not fully present, like he was somewhere else. He was anxious
and restless with a heavy, rattling breath. There were two of
us that shared hands on with him for three hours. The healing, wholing support of the Radiant energy brought deep
relaxation and peace to him and to us. He seemed ready to go
when we left.

"When I visited the next day, his breathing was sound-
less and quiet. It seemed he had recovered. At the beginning
of the session, he seemed worried, talked disjointedly and
moved his arm restlessly up and down. The hands-on session,
combined with calming words, bathed him again in deep
relaxation and peace.

"Subsequent visits provided him with the same deep peace,
but I noticed that his wife was getting more anxious so I
asked her how she was feeling.

"She shared that she was afraid and worried about the
future, wondering when and if he would die. I spent time with
her, gave her Attunements, and we did a session together.
She enjoyed it very much and felt more peaceful about her
husband. I reviewed with her ways she could continue to radiantly support herself and her husband. My heart filled with
radiant love for her and, when I left, she hugged me with gratitude. Later that day, I walked to a beautiful park and rested
on a bench beside a little pond facing the colourful leaves of

the trees and feeling the warm sun on my face. I gently placed my hands on my heart and began attuning the couple and his dying process. I experienced deeper love, compassion, gratitude and joy. Within this inner silence, I had a profound connection to light and life's continuum."

All Embracing Love

Maya Melrose, a Hospice social worker in South England, has studied to The Sixth Degree and is an Authorized Instructor of TRT®.

"My conscious journey with The Radiance Technique® began during my mother's dying process. We worked together to find ways to ease the process, and she experienced a sense of peace listening to the spring bird songs and reciting a simple mantra to help calm her mind. I was aware there was much more to be learnt about assisting someone through this important life transition and made an inner commitment to discover this knowledge.

"A few months after her death, I experienced intense grief, and a friend who had recently studied The First Degree Official Program of The Radiance Technique®, Authentic Reiki®, offered to give me a hands-on session for which I am eternally grateful. I felt nurtured by her gentle touch and amazed by how quickly my mood lifted and awareness expanded. I had found the doorway to the knowledge I was looking for and soon began my own studies of this profound transcendental science.

"Thirteen years later, I am working in a hospice where I am given an abundance of opportunities to use TRT to support patients, families and staff. Hospices were founded on the principle of helping people who are dying live as fully as possible, and TRT, with its life-enhancing and wholing qualities, combines naturally with all aspects of hospice care.

"On the wards, I inwardly pattern the cosmic symbols through all my interactions. I constantly use Radiant Touch®

with myself in Head Position #4 and Front Positions #1 and #3, and with patients, I gently hold their hands or lightly rest a hand on their arms connecting with their radiant heart centres. I have observed how many patients, when they are at rest, lie with one hand on their own heart centre.

"At other times, I direct energy in my office using the Attunement processes and at our noon quiet time for staff to expand the Radiant energy field for everyone in the hospice.

"Many patients come to us for the relief of pain and other symptoms and then return home. In my role as a social worker, I help arrange their care at home; patterning cosmic symbols, keeping my hands-on Head Position #4 and Front Position #1 while I make phone calls and discuss their needs helps to facilitate and reassure. I spend time with relatives on the wards, and hands-on Back Position #1 can be comforting and non-intrusive.

"When visiting bereaved relatives at home, I direct attunements and use Front Positions #1, #2 and #3 on myself while listening to them express their feelings and talk about the person who has died.

"As part of my working day, I also have the joy of giving hands-on sessions to staff and volunteers. Three staff members who are TRT® alumni offer half hour sessions and TRT® has become well established in the staff support system. Nurses and other staff have commented on feeling nurtured, and are surprised at how quickly they are able to unwind after a busy shift.

"I feel supported always by TRT® as I move through the day, and knowing that I will be able to recharge and renew in my transcendental meditation using TRT® Hands-on after work has been invaluable in stressful situations. During these meditations, I can feel my cells letting go of the demands of the day, and the stillness and inner peace is deeply refreshing after the intensity of relating in a hospice environment. Simultaneously, I am able to use the attunement processes within TRT® on the inner planes, and now I have a technique that has no time or space limitations in its application. I am able to continue to inner-connect when people have made their transition. This is a deep honour. My heart continues to open to the point of light within all living beings and the knowingness that death is a profound and significant life event.

"When I studied The Second Degree, discovering how to direct radiant energy on a timeless continuum to my mother in her transition process and doing this on an ongoing basis as I have advanced in my study of TRT® was deeply healing. I am celebrating the mystery of living as a human being each day, being able to use this cosmic science to bring more Radiant Light into our lives on planet earth and to hold the dying in the energy of All Embracing Love."

Maya's sharing is a clear example demonstrating how Radiant energy is generated from a Point of Light within and is not limited by distance or time. Having TRT® supports and expands our caregiving on deeper levels and our capacity for real compassion.

1 Barbara Ray, Ph.D., *The Expanded Reference Manual of The Radiance Technique®*, Authentic Reiki®, (St. Petersburg, FL: Radiance Associates, 1992), p. 116.

The Prayer of St. Francis

Lord make me an instrument of Your peace;
where there is hatred, let me sow love;
where there is injury, pardon;
where there is doubt, faith;
where there is despair, hope;
where there is darkness, light;
and where there is sadness, joy.
O Divine Master, grant that I may
not so much seek to be consoled as to console;
to be understood, as to understand;
to be loved, as to love;
for it is in giving that we receive,
it is in pardoning that we are pardoned,
and it is in dying that we are born to eternal life.

~ St. Francis of Assisi

Nursing Companions

*As a nurse, I am empowered
not by 'controlling' everything,
but rather by 'interacting' with
any situation that presents itself.
Radiant Touch® gives me the power
to interact with my patient,
no matter the status.
Radiant Touch® supports
my patients silently, deeply,
more than any outer gesture
I could do by itself.*

*~ Leslie Christopher, Women's Health Nurse Practitioner
Authorized Instructor of The Radiance Techique®*

-6-

THE VALUE OF HUMAN TOUCH has made a comeback in nursing care, and this chapter explores how nurses are using The Radiance Technique® both professionally and personally. In palliative care, old and new ways of care are re-emerging as the concept of the "whole person" is recognized and embraced. The following experiences from Canadian, British and American nurses speak for themselves; even when a cure is no longer an option, TRT®is an invaluable resource at the touch of a nurse's hand.

At The Hospice of Windsor and Essex County, nurse educators are part of a care team of consultants with specialized knowledge and expertise in cancer and other life-threatening illnesses. They counsel and teach patients and families how to address the physical, psychological, spiritual and social aspects of their disease.

Over the years the Hospice nursing team have incorporated The Radiance Technique® into their clinical practice and have found TRT®to be an invaluable tool to address both physical and emotional needs.

Invaluable Tool

"Whether the challenge be the fear and anxiety of patients experiencing chemotherapy for the first time, an acute pain episode, dealing with everyday uncertainties of a life-threatening illness or facilitating the transition to a peaceful death, The Radiance Technique® has been an invaluable tool for us to use throughout our patients' and families' journeys with their illnesses. It has been the constant intervention we can use when there is nothing else to do," writes Nurse Educator June James, R.N.

June, a founding member of Hospice and the first nurse at Hospice, shares the following experiences of using TRT® on the job:

"I had been following Michael, a 75-year-old man with cancer of the prostate with bone metastasis, for some time. He came into the hospital in a pain crisis with bone metastasis and metabolic problems which caused him to be very confused and agitated.

"After advocating with nursing staff to have an analgesic given, I went into the room where he lay writhing in bed, moaning, calling out and fighting to get out of bed.

"Several family members were present, all trying to calm him and prevent him from crawling out of bed. I plugged in my soothing music, spoke to him softly and gently placed my hands on Front Position #1. Within a few moments, his restlessness stopped, and he closed his eyes. I explained to the family what I was doing, and then, using the symbols I learned in The Second Degree, I directed energy to the family. When the analgesic finally started to work, I met with the family to address their many questions about the 'magic' in my hands that brought such fast, dramatic relief.

"I have numerous experiences I could relate about TRT®. So many times, I have found it so helpful: when a colleague has a headache, when a caregiver is sobbing uncontrollably and wants to regain control, when a patient is being admitted in a panic state about a new symptom, when I am stressed by too much to do and not enough time, The Radiance Technique® is the one constant that is always readily available and always helps."

Natural Pain Release

Although The Radiance Technique® is not a medical treatment for disease or symptom removal, a natural pain-release can follow the soothing application of hands-on. Documentation indicates when the body relaxes, the natural endorphins known as the body's natural painkillers are released.[1] Pain is especially common in advanced cancers and can affect a person's mood, sleep, activities and quality of life immensely. Pain can be continuous or intermittent. No one wants to see a loved one uncomfortable, and TRT® provides a gentle comforting support of gradual balance within the person.

It is helpful to understand the cycles of pain when giving sessions and to ask patients how they are feeling in that moment. Listening ears and watchful eyes help guide you. Physical pain can be described as nociceptive and neuropathic. Professionals define nociceptive pain in two types: somatic and visceral. Somatic pain is muscular or bone pain which has qualities of aching, deep dull throbbing. A more superficial level is localized to the skin with burning, itching or prickly feeling. Visceral pain involves visceral organs like the GI tract and pancreas with qualities of a constant deep pressure and stabbing pain. Neuropathic pain has qualities of burning, aching and severe pain from even slight pressure from clothing or light touch.[2] Knowing about these physical characteristics and how your patient feels helps you to be sensitive to their needs and enables you to direct the Radiant energy where additional support might be needed. TRT® helps alleviate physical discomfort and works well in conjunction with pain medications, often lengthening the periods of pain relief. Pain is not limited to the physical and on this subject, Dr. Barbara Ray offers the following insight:

> *Pain — Suffering or distress in any plane of body, emotion or mind. For releasing, balancing and transforming painful energy according to your individual process, use various*

aspects of The Radiance Technique® for as long and as often as you choose. Pain is an important signal that some energy is off-balance or blocked. The Radiance Technique® also facilitates your getting in touch with and releasing blocked pain patterns which are keeping you from natural growth and opening. Use in appropriate positions and, for extended time in meditating, use Head Positions #1, #2 and #3, Front Positions #1, #3 and #4 and Back Position #3.[3]

Providing adequate pain control is at the forefront of palliative care and combining TRT® gives the patient an opportunity to experience a higher quality of life and inner peace. In addition to a complete twelve-position session, spending extra time in painful areas can make a considerable difference in the control of pain, and in special cases, hands are held above the area of the body, not even touching the clothing. Practitioners can use various aspects of TRT® in this case as well. In particular, Head Position #2 is especially helpful for pain release. In the following, a nurse describes how the simplicity and ease of TRT® benefits both the giver and receiver for natural pain release.

Carole Jones, R.N., assists Palliative Care Physicians in the Windsor Regional Cancer Centre's Pain Clinic. Carole's Radiant hands come to the aid of many who pass through the Clinic's door. "One afternoon, the radiation technicians felt helpless as a 41-year-old man with advanced lung cancer screamed in pain as they transferred him from the ambulance stretcher to the radiation table," Carole recalls. "While he was on the table, I placed my hands in sequence on all four Head Positions for the next 30 minutes. The staff was so grateful. Bill's anxiety and breathing pattern changed after ten minutes, and the pain began to subside after 20 minutes. Along with his breakthrough Dilaudid medication and Radiant Touch®, Bill was able to relax, become more peaceful and have his radiation treatment for pain relief."

Supporting a Peaceful Journey

Carole also shares this personal experience of her colleague and friend diagnosed with advanced breast cancer:

"Jennie was a fun-loving registered nurse in her early 50s who delivered quality care to her patients and had a passion for life. She had received sessions of Radiant Touch® while on her chemotherapy, and we had often talked of the relaxing and calming effect it gave her. She completed a difficult course of chemotherapy and radiation, only to develop distant metastasis requiring a bone marrow transplant and further high dose chemotherapy in the hopes of living.

"The bone marrow transplant failed and the high dose of chemo caused permanent kidney and liver damage, and Jennie was intubated and placed on a respirator. For some time, I felt helpless when her family made the decision to remove life support. The tube in her throat was removed and the respirator turned off. Jennie's colour became ashen and her heart slowed. I thought that at least I could offer her Radiant Touch®. I placed my hands on her heart centre as the family encircled the bed. After 15 minutes, I changed to Front Position #2 for ten minutes, but found improved colour and peacefulness with Front Position #1 and moved my hands back to her heart centre. Before, I would have felt hopeless, but with my training in TRT®, I supported Jeannie through her dying. I gave the family hope that someone was doing something while her life was ending. Radiantly supporting Jennie in the last few moments of her life gave her peace, her family peace and myself peace. The Radiant energy of TRT® allows me to be more compassionate and nurturing and makes me a better nurse, especially in cases where there is no hope for cure. I can still do something that provides personal support."

One of the amazing interactions of Radiant energy is its support for a peaceful transition. Carole, her friend and family received that benefit after making the difficult decision to

take her off the respirator. TRT®opened the door for experiencing the gift of peace in the moments of transition. Often
people will feel a sense of helplessness in these circumstances.
As Dr. Barbara Ray writes:

Helplessness/Powerlessness — *The Radiance Technique®*
offers a unique and profound tool to help in restoring a sense
of well-being, balance and inner power to a person going
through any situation, condition or circumstance which
tends to evoke feelings of helplessness and powerlessness. You
can help yourself and others to restore themselves to a sense
of well-being and wholeness, even when difficult decisions
are necessary, and in the situations of severe and/or life-
threatening diseases whether physical or psychological...[4]

Waiting to Exhale

Nurses continue to express how their traditional medical
training and medical interventions are limited, and how
grateful they are to have a tool like The Radiance Technique®
to offer support that extends beyond the physical. Alison
Sherwood, R.N., shares about her first experience with a
dying patient. "My sense of helplessness was profound. The
family's anxiety and grief, together with the patient's struggle,
was felt in my chest like a pulling sensation. I asked the family if I could try a relaxation technique that I had just learned,
and with their permission, I placed my hands on Front
Position #1, the heart centre. With this first experience, I
noted the patient's respirations relaxed and slowed, and the
patient calmed. His face looked relaxed and less stressed. Of
course, as these changes occurred, the family relaxed as well,
and I felt myself calming; my breathing slowed and my heartbeat was less pronounced in my chest. Over a short period of
time, this patient died, quietly and peacefully. The family was
grateful and comforted that their loved one had passed on.

I felt peaceful in helping in this transition, and my sense of grief was lessened.

"This first very positive experience with TRT® used in the dying process was certainly very rewarding for me, and I have since used it in many similar situations. Practicing TRT® on my patients near the time of their death has been a very intimate sharing with them. It is like a final gift we share together and a way to say 'thank you and good-bye.'

"I have also been able to use TRT® to support myself not only with a full session for relaxation, stress and clearing my mind, but also as a short stress reliever. Often during a stressful day dealing with patient issues, I may find myself rushing from one crisis to another. During these times, I notice my heart rate is elevated, my breathing more short and shallow, my thinking less clear and my anxiety high. While driving in my car from one patient to another, I place one hand over my heart centre while trying to refocus. With this, I find my breathing slowing and becoming deeper; I become calmer and by the time I reach my next appointment, I am calmer and my thinking is clearer. At other times, by using the heart centre and the solar plexus positions, I can also calm myself before a meeting or a personal diagnostic test."

Expanding Plan of Care

For many years, Shelley Dobson, R.N., has worked in hospital, Hospice and community environments and has integrated TRT® into her care planning:

"As a nurse of 28 years, 27 of which I was not aware of The Radiance Technique®, I have found countless opportunities for its use, both for my personal life and with my patients and their families.

"I have found that when I sit with a family who is struggling to make a decision about something that has never presented itself in their lives before, I place one hand on my heart, take a deep breath and then wait momentarily. I am then able to help these families in a calm and thoughtful manner, discuss with them possible treatment plans, end of life plans and even future plans. More often than I can count, the individual with the life-threatening illness responds quickly to me. The panic in the eyes of patients lessens as they hear someone who seems to understand them and their position with family members, who may not yet be aware or accepting of existing and imminent changes.

"I use my hands-on during telephone conversations with patients, families and other team members when I need to use the most appropriate language to obtain the desired results for all involved.

"Personally, on sleepless nights, I am able to use the Front Positions, and sleep seems to follow a bit more easily.

"I have used Radiant Touch® with my mother and not only watched her become more relaxed but observed our relationship taken to a different level of understanding.

"I have always *lived in the moment*, but now I am even more observant of life and all living things around me. So, as a nurse who once believed we only saved lives through acute medical intervention, I am now able to see the benefit of applying both acute and complementary interventions together in a proposed plan of care."

Self-Renewal

Applying TRT® in patient care is beneficial on so many levels, and nurses using it in self care find that it provides energy restoring and revitalizing benefits. Louise Grant, R.N., describes using TRT® at the end of her day for self-renewal:

"I have a rewarding but very challenging job as a nurse in a hospice for the dying in Devon, UK. After doing hands-on in bed following a very stressful day at work, the day seemed to disappear. All my worries went away, and I fell into a wonderful sleep. I had to be up for another shift early in the morning but awoke feeling very refreshed and ready to face another day. Since studying TRT®, I feel able to cope with anything, knowing that I can go home and relax with my Radiant Touch®."

Caring Heart and Hands in the E.R.

Diana Davis Robinson, R.N., worked for 40 years in the Windsor area as nurse. Her most recent position was Director of the Patient Unit for the Emergency/Trauma at Hotel-Dieu Grace hospital. Now retired, Diana explains how TRT® supported her as well as her patients:

"Nursing was my passion. I have had the privilege to touch and make a difference in people's lives in ways no one else can understand or imagine from birth to death.

"In May 1995 I received The First Degree Official Program in The Radiance Technique®, Authentic Reiki® during training for our team of hospital nursing directors. Immediately, I applied it on myself every day to balance, support and keep my thoughts organized to assist me in prioritizing my day. Most days were long and stressful not only with the E.R. itself, but with the array of administrative duties including reports, schedules, budgets and meetings. The hands-on allowed me to support myself whenever necessary, no matter where or when. All I needed was my hands to assist me to be calm, cool and collected.

"About two months after my class, I arrived at work earlier than usual to touch base with the night shift going off duty. They were upset because one of the patients, a fellow nurse, was dying with cancer, and she had been in pain all night. Even with a morphine drip and injections to support the infusion, she remained restless and in pain. The family had been there all night and the E.R. physician and staff were having trouble coping with being unable to comfort her. They asked if I had any ideas. I said I would go and speak with the patient and family. While walking to the patient's room, I wondered if what I had learned in class would really work. After introducing myself to Lynn and her family, I explained what TRT® was and asked for their permission to use it in an effort to make Lynn more comfortable. They were skeptical but agreed, for they had run out of options. I suggested that the family to go and have some breakfast and coffee in the cafeteria and come back in about 1½ hours. The youngest daughter wanted to stay close by and that was fine with me. I described to Lynn what I was going to do and informed her that she could ask me to stop anytime she wished. In that time, Lynn shared with me that she was ready to die but was worried about her family, as they did not want to let her go. I asked her if she wanted me to speak with her family, and she gently nodded.

"For the next hour, I began hands-on. Lynn's breathing eased and became deep and regular. Her whole body relaxed, and she drifted off into a deep sleep and so did her daughter. I waited outside her room for the family to return and shared with them that Lynn was ready to make her transition. I was worried about leaving them and wanted to make sure that they would be okay. In the hallway, they began to share more of their feelings. I asked them to give Lynn permission to die and assure her that they would be okay. And they did.

"Amazed at how peaceful she looked, the family wanted to know what drug I had given her. I smiled, showing my hands and shared that I used Radiant Touch® with her. Lynn expressed to everyone that it was the first time in a long time that she felt no pain and was totally at peace.

"A half-hour later, staff moved Lynn to a medical floor. Then about an hour later, the family came back to the E.R. to thank me. Lynn had made her transition, pain-free, alert and able to communicate with them prior to her death. I felt privileged to support and to assist in her transition. I have since used TRT® on other patients, family members, my dogs, and plants and continue to use TRT® everyday on myself. It gives me a peaceful calm and a clear head. I feel TRT® should be part of a nurse's curriculum to aid him or her in caring for their patients. I love nursing and using TRT because it allows me to use my gift of caring with my head, heart and hands."

Calming Touch at the Beside

Bonnie Atmore, R.N., with The Second Degree, uses TRT® in short intervals while at her desk writing patient reports and during difficult phone calls. She also shares Radiant Touch® with her patients and recalls an 80-year-old patient with advanced osteoporosis. "Caroline's mobility was severely limited because of her advanced disease status," she explains. "In January 1999, she was admitted to the hospital for investigations. She sustained a fall, fracturing her hip. Her fragile status was such that surgery was not performed. Narcotics were required to control pain. Caroline became confused, agitated and aggressive from the prolonged use of the analgesic. Family and staff were not able to calm or soothe her. She would have no recollection of family or friends being at her bedside.

"I had been giving her sessions of Radiant Touch® at home prior to this admission. I continued to do so in the hospital setting. During her agitation, I was able to do Head Positions #1 and #2 and Front Position #1. She would calm down during the ten to 15-minute sessions.

"Caroline remained in this state for four weeks before returning to her former placid self. Once herself again, she was able to share with us that she had virtually no recall of that four week period. She did acknowledge, however, her awareness of the times she was receiving Radiant Touch®, for she felt calmer and had an awareness of my presence. She attributes the ongoing TRT® sessions as being instrumental in getting through that most difficult time."

Transforming with Dying

The soothing hands-on of Radiant Touch® is an enormous support for patients experiencing fear, pain and respiratory distress. The sense of calm, peace and final release that can be experienced is expressed eloquently in the following sharing from Lynda Lang, R.N., with The Second Degree:

"In 1994, about a month after I completed The First Degree Official Program of The Radiance Technique®, Authentic Reiki®, I arrived at a patient's home who was in the final stage of cancer. I found myself in the midst of chaos. Jack, whom I had been visiting for the last couple of months, was in a severe respiratory crisis, sitting forward in his armchair, colour ashen, eyes wide with panic, his stridorous, crowing respirations audible on the front porch. His son and wife were crying and pacing, having exhausted all the possibilities: pain meds were given, anti-anxiety meds, oxygen, and yet no relief. Feeling at a loss to offer any further medical solution for the time being, I offered to try a relaxation technique, and the family agreed.

"I placed my hands on Head Position #1 and proceeded through the various positions, allowing three to five minutes for each, though it seemed more like ten minutes. I immediately noticed a slowing in his respiratory rate and a lessening of the harsh, crowing inspirations which distressed everyone in the room.

"Eventually, his eyes closed and with gentle coaxing, Jack was able to sit back in his chair, giving the impression of some relief from his pain. The family members were awestruck and sat at his side holding his hands, softly crying and urging me to continue.

"As we all watched, I continued with the Front Positions, making adjustments as necessary for his slumped posture, our eyes fixed on his face and chest movements. An aura of peace and tranquility settled over us. Jack breathed quietly, and the deep lines in his face seemed to relax. Some colour flushed his cheeks, and we all took an easier breath.

"It was becoming apparent to me that an amazing transformation was happening here, and I pointed out to the family the changes I was seeing, and they nodded in agreement. The respirations grew quieter, less frequent and shallower, and his neck and shoulder muscles relaxed.

"Eventually, the respirations ceased entirely, and we were breathless ourselves to see the serene expression on his face. The family were beyond tears at this point as they had never expected such a beautiful ending to such a long, distressing illness full of pain and burdensome symptoms.

"We all felt spiritually bonded and honoured to be present at this death. It was difficult to explain to others what had exactly transpired; the special feeling seemed diminished when translating it into mere words.

"I think about this experience often, grateful for the gift of The Radiance Technique® and how it supported me as a caregiver in a difficult situation. I realize now it was an invaluable tool to facilitate the transition of an individual through the dying process."

Lynda's sharing was a real experience of inner connection. TRT® allows those who assist the dying person to connect on a profound level as Dr. Barbara Ray writes:

> The momentous occasion of death represents a truly cosmic happening as the Soul continues on its journey into new dimensions. The Radiance Technique® gives you a powerful yet gentle and harmless way of participating without intruding, of touching life, not death, and of experiencing Oneness, not separateness, with yourself or with another going through this profound process. [5]

When offering hands-on support, one can be in all types of environments as mentioned earlier: giving hands-on before radiation treatments while on a table, in chairs and among medical equipment, pumps and drips. The key is to be flexible, and having training in degrees beyond The First Degree can open up more possibilities of support for others and for self. Any amount of TRT® is supportive and transformative.

Silent Support from Within

Leslie Christopher, MN, WHNP, a Women's Health Nurse Practitioner with the United States Air Force, has studied to The Seventh Degree and shares her experience of supporting a patient in the final moments of her life:

"One of my patients was an elderly woman who was unconscious and on a ventilator. She had been intubated despite a 'Do Not Resuscitate' order. The family was upset. Once someone has been intubated with mechanical ventilation, it is not an easy thing to stop. No one wants to take the responsibility, and a political quagmire often ensues. Doctors, family and hospital administration heatedly discussed the policies involved and paperwork needed to remove her from the ventilator.

"While all the chaos swirled around the patient, I continued to care for her. I applied Radiant Touch® to her and directed Cosmic Symbols to the situation. Even when unconscious, TRT® can support the point of wholeness deep within the patient.

"Despite numerous machines and even the dying process, I had no feelings of helplessness or powerlessness. As a nurse, I am empowered not by 'controlling' everything, but rather by 'interacting' with any situation that presents itself. Radiant Touch® gives me the power to interact with my patient, no matter the status. Radiant Touch® supports my patients silently, deeply, more than any outer gesture I could do by itself."

In the circle of care, nurses are often the first individuals to offer comfort, understanding and support to people facing a life-threatening illness. They are often at the bedside until the very end of life providing compassionate support through this passage. Extending their hands and generating Radiant Light energy enriches their lives and those in their care.

[1] Barbara Ray, Ph.D., *The Official Handbook of The Radiance Technique®, Authentic Reiki®*, (St. Petersburg, FL: The Radiance Technique International Association, Inc., and Radiance Seminars, Inc., 1984), p. 22.

[2] The Windsor-Essex End of Life Steering Committee, *The Erie St. Clair Palliative Care Management Tools*, January 2007, 3rd Edition Version 3.1, Pain Classification & Description, p. 34.

[3] Barbara Ray, Ph.D., *The Expanded Reference Manual of The Radiance Technique®, Authentic Reiki®*, (St. Petersburg, FL: Radiance Associates, 1987), p. 83

[4] *Ibid.*, p. 50.

[5] Barbara Ray, Ph.D., *The 'Reiki' Factor in The Radiance Technique® Expanded Edition*, (St. Petersburg, FL: Radiance Associates, 1992), p. 103

PART 4

May the long-time sun shine upon you,
All love surround you,
And the pure light within you,
Guide your way home.

~ Traditional Blessing

The Passage in Light

*...With The Radiance Technique® you can have the
honor of assisting as the soul departs
its 'connection' to that particular body.
It is a profound realization 'to know' that
death is not a disease, is not a negative
and is not the end of all but rather is a
significant and meaningful process
within Life and in polarity with birth.
In one of its deepest, inner aspects
The Radiance Technique®
is an ancient science of Light
derived from and related to the
Egyptian Mystery of the Passage into Light (mis-
named The Egyptian Book of the Dead) and the
transition processes of the ancient Tibetan passage
into Life Eternal
(Tibetan Book of the Dead).*[1]

*~ Dr. Barbara Ray, Ph.D
The Expanded Reference Manual of
The Radiance Technique®, Authentic Reiki®*

-7-

THE MYSTERY OF THE JOURNEY OF DYING, the final move within, begins at what is known, the physical deterioration of the body, to what is unknown. But is it unknown? Ancient texts, scriptures and oral transmissions reveal knowledge of those who have explored worlds beyond the gates of death. People with near-death experiences have come back to reveal some of the mysteries in their own words. Numerous people tell of seeing light. Entering these inner worlds using The Radiance Technique® can bring us to a point where the outer world is temporarily suspended — the pain, the racing thoughts, the fear as we connect to the inner and are held in the vibrational energy of Radiant Light, a time where the two worlds begin to merge together as transition gets closer. As nurses shared in the previous chapter, supporting someone with TRT® during the final stages of life opens the gateway to help one die more peacefully. TRT® does not cross natural order, but instead supports a person's natural process, balancing all the outer and inner levels of being. This chapter continues to explore how TRT® supports this natural transition we will all some day experience.

The hospice movement around the world has brought consciousness and contemplation about death and dying to the forefront, and there are many books, videos, courses and organizations devoted to this cycle of our lives. Dr. Jane Buckle, Ph.D., R.N., has worked for many years in palliative care and writes about the physical experiences in her book, *Clinical Aromatherapy in Nursing*:

"The process of dying is recognizable. Bodily functions cease and the peripheral temperature drops as the circulation fails, leaving the skin mottled and discoloured. Thirst is often the last craving, with food refused. Many dying patients breathe through their mouths, which can become dry and cracked. Often their eyes are open even though they may be asleep or unconscious. Rattling in the throat occurs when secretions collect in the throat and the patient is too weak to cough." She continues, "Cheyne-Stoke breathing also often occurs prior to death. The patient may be aware that someone is with them, even though they appear to be deeply unconscious. It is recognized that hearing is the last sense to go, so what is said in front of a dying patient is important."[2]

Seeing Beyond the Skin

Death is not merely a medical event. We witness these outer manifestations, but can we see beyond the physical boundaries? Do we really survive our own physical death? Death is so difficult for many in our Western culture because we have identified most of our lives with our outer form, not with our wholeness. For some, death is seen as an end; for some, a beginning; and for others, a continuation. Knowing we are much more than our body can allow us to have less fear about death. In a summer retreat, one of my teachers, Gelek Rimpoche, shared, "Our knowledge and views are so limited, we still see life as birth to death; we cannot see beyond. We don't have a panoramic view, we have a sandwiched view."[3]

With TRT®, we can begin to understand our multi-dimensions beyond the capacity of our mental mind, beyond having a belief. We have the capacity to touch these levels of ourselves that are present here and now and continue on long after we have vacated our physical home. Application of TRT® connects us with our true nature and on this theme, Dr. Barbara Ray sheds some light:

Eternal — *Refers to the principle of energy which is "forever"* — *which is "always"* — *an energy of the inner planes of your Being* — *the inner energies of the soul and especially of Pure Spirit, Real Light. The Radiance Technique® is a cosmic science accessing universal energy which has the inner quality and radiance of "forever," of "eternal"* — <u>*beyond*</u> *the limits and qualities of partial energies of limited (according to their energy principle) non-enduring planes of reality.*[4]

Ganga Stone's book, *Start the Conversation*, is based on her workshops which focus on helping others understand death and appreciate life. "Fear and grief are the thieves of joy — and of any hope of joy. Yet they rest on a single simple but false assumption — that the human being is only a body, a mere thing — and that the entire being is destroyed with the body at death. On this tragically mistaken belief rests all the suffering — all the grief and all the fear — that make it so difficult to live out a life of whatever duration, in freedom and in joy."[5]

Living and dying are profound. What is happening physically is not all that is happening. This time of transition is extremely subtle, and what is happening is not tangible. Richard Gerber, M.D., and author of *A Practical Guide to Vibrational Medicine*, shares his expanded view of death:

"The issue of death and spiritual energy also helps highlight the way the vibrational-medicine model differs from the existing mechanistic paradigm of healing. Seen from the mechanistic viewpoint, the human brain and body are merely a collection of chemicals, energized and animated by electrical and electrochemical impulses. To the purely mechanistic thinkers, death means the end of the body as well as the destruction of the personality. But in the vibrational or energetic model, spirit is seen as the motivating force that animates the physical form. That is, our spirit, like a vaporous ghost, inhabits the mechanical vehicle we call the physical body. At time of death, our spirit moves on, leaving behind only a life-less shell. In the vibrational-medicine model, it is the beingness of our spirit and its experiential journey through the physical world that creates the real adventure and mystery of a person's life."[6]

Experiences with clients have led me to this deep inner knowledge. Gelek Rimpoche, one of the last reincarnated lamas to be trained in Tibet, writes about the process of dying in his book *Good Life, Good Death*, "The time of dying is a very sensitive period. We're dissolving, withdrawing from all our senses, from our fingers, hands, arms, limbs. We are retreating, retreating, retreating, until finally we retreat even from the seed we collected from our parents, into our deepest point. Our sensitivities become extremely heightened now."[7]

To be by someone's side and support their journey, as Rimpoche describes, has left lasting imprints within me. Sheila was one of my clients who had a profound effect on my life, my work, giving me a raison d'être, and encouraging me to learn deeper aspects of myself. I experienced that being with dying is about living. In her final moments, Sheila connected to a peace and freedom she never thought possible.

A Healing Transformation

Sheila, like many other patients I have known, sought alternatives as current traditional medicine could offer her no more treatments. At age 58, she received the diagnosis of ovarian cancer that had spread to her lungs and liver. This was not a good prognosis. A university professor, Sheila was highly intelligent and open to trying new things, and so a referral for her from a Hospice nurse was made, and we began our journey together with TRT®.

I remember clearly the fall day that she came to see me. We marvelled at the beautiful leaves on the trees outside the Radiant Touch® room windows. Then, she began talking to me about preparing for death. She was scared; she felt the unknown strongly. And then she asked me something, something no one had ever asked me before. She said, "Christine, I want you to help me die."

I remember that moment. As our gaze penetrated to a deeper level, I felt myself tingle in my body. Time stood still. Silence. This was what Oprah Winfrey would call a magic moment, remembering your spirit. What an honour. I had silently supported many people before, but never had someone consciously asked me this way.

So we began.

Sheila was amazed that her sessions of TRT® could bring her to a peaceful place. I shared with her my journey of cancer, and we connected even more on a deeper level.

It seemed like overnight Sheila became weaker and her ability to focus for long periods of time became shorter and shorter. I did not have a TRT® class scheduled for another month. I was not sure if she could sit through one anyway, given her rapid physical decline, so I began to teach Sheila privately over the next four weeks The First Degree Official Program of The Radiance Technique®, Authentic Reiki®. Even wheelchair-bound and on oxygen, she came for her classes. During this time, she also attended a group called *Exploring My Dying* offered at The Hospice Wellness Centre. This group supports and challenges individuals to become more comfortable with dying, to talk about it, name it and learn that exploring dying is a part of ones' living. With the help of TRT®, we began to integrate some of the issues that the group brought up for her in a wholistic way. In this process, we became each other's teacher.

Sheila felt TRT® assisted her on many levels. "TRT® redoes your proportionalities," she once said. "I am aware of how much of my mind space is taken up with my physical disease, yet many positive things are happening to me at the same time."

Sheila felt that her greatest challenge was her mind. She

had lived in her mind for so much of her life, and now she noticed that it caused her problems: "I can have all these negative thoughts, and thoughts of things I need to do, and get caught up in physical problems, and then by the end of the session, my mind changes. TRT® introduces other things supportive and pleasurable to me like the spiritual aspect. This is a really big plus for me."

Sheila discovered how much more there was within herself; she connected with her wholeness. She marvelled about "the idea of tapping into the centre of myself with my hands, seeing that I am light, universal light within. Most systems I know take the light in, but don't say it is already within you."

Her physical problems increased, and her physical appearance became noticeably thinner since she was already slender at six feet tall. More fluid began to collect in her lungs, lowering her lung capacity, increasing her pain and requiring weekly draining at the Cancer Centre. She began to question how much she was willing to go through. She said, "TRT® checks my runaway thoughts and brings me to the point of sleep which I find quite amazing. It is also helpful in quieting my stomach and head. When I have the combination of unable to breath and crazy belly, I put one hand on each Front Positions #1 and #3, and it helps tremendously."

Sheila summed up The Radiance Technique® as assisting her to reach the following:

"Time to feel peace.
Time to feel ready.
Time to make the next step by myself.
Time to let things go."

It was now the cold months of winter, and I began visiting Sheila at home, as she became confined to her bed. I believe people decide when they will die, and I knew that Sheila would also do this. During the last few sessions of TRT®, she could feel her fear and anxiety about dying rising. Sheila said she was not ready yet, and I assured her that she would only go when she was ready.

One Saturday evening, as I was driving along the Detroit River to her house, I felt an inner knowingness that this would be my final session with her. From far away, I could see the clouds in the sky open, and rays of light were streaming down. It was so magnificent it reminded me of one of those photographs of light with religious significance. One part of me did not want to see it, it was so beautiful. My own fears began to surface. As I drove closer to her home, the light was shining directly above her house. It was amazing. This was it. I knew it. As I parked my car, I took a few moments to close my eyes and give myself an Attunement. I was not sure what the fear I had was all about, and I spent a few more minutes with my hands on my heart. As I stepped out of the car, I patterned Cosmic Symbols. As I met her husband and son, I patterned. I continued to pattern up the stairs to her room.

I walked quietly into her room and sat in the chair beside her bed. Even her room looked different today. She surrounded herself with beauty. Many vases of flowers filled the room, her favourite classical music, Mozart's *Wish for Spring*, was playing softly, and even the labels on her bottles of medication were covered up (as she told me later, to avoid distracting herself from creating a healing space). Sheila slowly opened her eyes and said to me, "I am ready. I am finally ready." I felt my fear leaving. She began to tell me of her deep and profound experience that had happened two nights earlier during her hands-on. I asked her if it was okay if I wrote down what she said and quickly got out a pen and some paper from my purse.

"She said the girl is beautiful
But she said she is blind.
She said the girl has a shovel
But she said she had no soil.

This went on and on, no way out of this intellectual turmoil, the little girl was me. Finally, the girl experienced a release, an awakening and she experienced light. She made it through it all, and now finally she feels free.

Now her eyes — she only sees
She feels the light, senses it.
Her body may be ugly, have problems, but she feels free, feels peaceful."

I was utterly amazed. I wrote very quickly even though I wanted to just be there listening without writing, but something told me this was important. She had experienced what I had read about — Radiant clarity of the nature of her mind. She actualized freedom from the darkness of all the distractions of her mental plane. She was able to dissolve them by being supported by Radiant transcendental Light.

I remember reading earlier an excerpt in *The Tibetan Book of Living and Dying* by Sogyal Rinpoche, "As the body dies, the senses and subtle elements dissolve, and this is followed by the death of the ordinary aspect of our mind, with all its negative emotions of anger, desire and ignorance. Finally, nothing remains to obscure our true nature, as everything that in life has clouded the enlightened mind has fallen away. And what is revealed is the primordial ground of our absolute nature, which is like a pure and cloudless sky."[8]

I asked her if there was anyone she needed to call or speak to, and Sheila said she had already made her last calls overseas earlier that morning. Sheila shared that she had asked her son to stay home from university until Tuesday, and requested her husband to take the next week off from work. Yes, she knew when she was going to die. She had it planned.

Our time together that evening was a gift to me beyond words. As I began patterning, everything in the room became "light-filled." The Cosmic Symbols provided a gateway on the inner planes to connect to and experience this expanded Radiant Universal Light.

We began sharing a session. Sheila sat up in bed and was able to hold her hands on Front Positions #3 and #4. I started with the Head Positions, and every fifteen minutes I soaked a small sponge in water and applied it to her dry lips. She pursed her lips to get every single drop of water. That evening, I continually patterned Cosmic Symbols for our entire time together, connecting from the highest vibrational point of light within me to the highest vibrational point of light within Sheila.

I had been with people before supporting their transition, but this experience was different. Sheila was aware and conscious of her dying, and she had been using TRT® on herself. She journeyed towards her transition consciously, choosing her time to let go and in her special way, ensuring everything was in order to make things easier for everyone else.

And then speaking ceased. After one and a half hours, she just stared straight ahead. I felt she was seeing things I was not able to see. She smiled now and then but did not talk anymore. I felt a deep love inside myself to be witness to such a mystery. I felt a deep celebration with Sheila's being and freedom. I sang and hummed again and again the following song, *Go now in beauty, peace be with you, 'til we meet again in the light.* Tears of joy streamed down my cheeks in celebration of this mysterious passage of death, this mystery of light, this interconnection to all that was, all that is and all that will be.

I did not want to leave, but I knew her family and friends needed to be with her. I directed one last Attunement in the presence of Sheila and patterned a Cosmic Symbol over each of her chakras. After two hours, I went downstairs to let the family know that she had stopped talking and was in a coma.

That evening and the next day, I continued to connect with Sheila on the inner planes by directing Radiant energy to her. Two days later, I was in the middle of a Radiant Touch®

session with a caregiver, and all of a sudden, I felt her presence come to me. I saw her face smiling, and I knew at that moment that she had made her transition. Her best friend later told me that when she died, it was with a Radiant smile. What a humbling and honouring experience. There are no greater gifts than this.

I remember re-reading the entry "Coma" in *The Expanded Reference Manual of TRT®, Authentic Reiki®*, in reference to what had transpired during my last visit to Sheila. They were no longer words or concepts, but I now had new eyes to see with and an inner knowing from my personal experience.

> *Coma — You can safely use The Radiance Technique® with someone in a coma. You can also apply the hands-on positions, with extra time, as you choose, on Head #1, #2 and #3; Front #1, #2 and #3, and Back #3. Remember, The Radiance Technique® accesses the point of wholeness __within__ you and the other person. As an Inner Plane science, The Radiance Technique® allows support and contact in radiance with the soul and spiritual dimensions and interacts as a Guide of Light.*[9]

Many spiritual traditions speak to something beyond this physical existence. Native traditions speak of the cycle of birth and death as being a continuous circle. In the book, *Wisdom of the Elders*, Peter Knudtson and David Suzuki write that the Inuit who live in north-central Canada believe in the continuum that life goes on without end: "At death, the soul is not extinguished. It lives on to surface again in another organism, investing it with a sacred spark of vitality and consciousness."[10] Maori acknowledge the spiritual pathway of their ancestors who passed on into the veil of the world without end. In the Bible when one leaves the body, the connection between the body and spirit is called "the silver cord," — "...the silver cord be loosed, or the golden bowl be broken. ..."[11] Core teachings of Tibetan Buddhism speak of outer and inner dissolution of ourselves at time of death and afterlife.

The dissolution of the four elements of earth, water, fire and air that make up a human body is a gradual movement toward more subtle levels of consciousness. Gelek Rimpoche writes that after death, "What really travels is a very subtle continuation of us, some kind of very subtle mind, a subtle energy like air."[12]

Through the application of TRT® Hands-on or directing Radiant energy, one is able to support the dying to and through the subtle levels. Sogyal Rimpoche conveys that this successive dissolution "moves gradually toward the revelation of the very subtlest consciousness of all: the Ground Luminosity or Clear Light."[13] My experience with Sheila opened my consciousness to the possibility of dying into this Radiant Clear Light. Dr. Barbara Ray shares her insights on this ancient energy:

> *More than five thousand years ago, the Egyptians affirmed their knowledge of the immortality of human Consciousness. In The Book of the Dead, which the Egyptians actually called the Book of Coming Forth to Light, many levels of the life of the soul were described, and it was written, 'I am like the stars who know not weariness — I am upon the Boat of Millions of Years.'*
>
> *The inner knowledge about life and science was kept secret and hidden, revealed to only a few chosen initiates. But in the current New Age of humanity, the doors are being thrown open and the knowledge distributed to all of us.*[14]

Many students of TRT® express their gratitude that such a sacred ancient energy is available for us to use at this period in history.

Profound Spiritual Care

I had been radiantly supporting Marie with home visits for a year. She had a recurrence of breast cancer that had metastasized to her colon. She did not readily allow others outside her family to get close to her, but she was open to try Radiant Touch®. From our very first session together, I saw her inner glow, her compassion and passion she had for others and for life. Now in her 70s, Marie had to face one of the most difficult challenges ahead. Marie had spent her life as a caregiver both at home and at work. She had retired from nursing, and although she had always filled her life with adventure, her priorities were her family; her children and grandchildren were number one. Marie had an enthusiasm and energy for life that many claimed was incomparable.

After a few sessions, she asked me to teach her how to apply TRT® on herself. It always brought her peace and a sense of calm in her emotions and mind. Our Radiant Touch® sessions together gave her relief, supporting her during her pain and feelings of depression. The most profound quality Marie found in TRT® was the ability to connect to her spiritual self, a part of herself she knew was not ill or diseased. This was very important for her, and sometimes she was so moved by her experiences that she cried. I realized that what was most comforting was not trying to provide answers, but just to be there, to listen and give her a direct experience of her inner light.

Marie's body grew weaker, too weak to move on her own, too weak to hold her head up. She was feeling more and more out of control of her physical body. There was so much more that she wanted to do with her grandchildren, and she asked the questions, why me and why now? She moved from being afraid of dying to being afraid of living because her physical realities became increasingly more difficult and painful.

Over the weeks, our conversations contained fewer words. Her skin seemed like an intrusion over her bones, the skin so dry and weathered. I gently rubbed her back with my fingertips, only feeling the protrusion of each one of her ribs. I held her hand. I helped her move to different positions because her tailbone was so sore from sitting directly on her bone. Marie told me that she was ready to die. That was the first time she had said that to me. She always had hope before, and we were trying to help her make it to her grandson's bar mitzvah, now only a few weeks away. But something within her let go, and Marie did not want to fight anymore. She asked me to help her die.

One week later, Marie was another week weaker, another week thinner. She repeated to me, "I just want to die now. I want to go into a coma and die. I can't take it anymore." She had suffered a long time and now was experiencing increased nausea. She used a spoon and pressed it at the back of her throat to help her throw up.

Her eyes took on a glossy appearance, looking at me, but not looking at me — looking through me to another place and time, clear and beyond this earthly sphere. Her body was so tired, she would move in and out of sleep.

When we normally shared a session of hands-on, I would place my hands on Marie's Head Positions, and she would place her hands on her Front Positions, but one day they were outstretched as if she was waiting for deliverance or a healing. I repeated Cosmic Symbols over and over again, attuning her, her body, her mind, her emotions and her spirit. I moved with her to a deeper level of consciousness. Our interconnection felt different from other times, not in a physical sense, but something much deeper, something much more profound. A place of bliss, of no pain, no worry, I felt uplifted. We always had our sessions overlooking the water. That day, as I gazed out the expansive windows, a beautiful sign from nature appeared. Seven swans in flight landed right in front of us on the Detroit River between the ice floes, a rare sight for the month of February.

I had a deep inner connection with the Radiant energy that pulsated and spiralled through Marie, through me, around her and around me. I connected to something greater than me, but yet a part of me. I held her while she tried to vomit; I caressed her hands, all the time using cosmic symbols for support and healing on all levels of her being.

I returned the next afternoon to find her family had moved her to the bedroom. Now, Marie was unable to move or speak. Pain medication increased to intervals every three hours. As the Woodstock chimes hanging from the magnolia tree outside her window gently sounded, I felt that they were ringing in celebration as she proceeded closer to her transition.

For all her trials and tribulations, her pain and suffering both physical and mental, I supported Marie silently. There was an incredible stillness in her room. Her eyes closed, Marie's outer appearance was almost shocking in comparison to the day before. I had left my Tibetan Tingshaw bells at her home for the past few weeks because she loved the sound they made. They were on the table beside her bed.

Family members shared final words and many tears. It was very honouring to be by her side as family spoke of their love for her and all that she had done. Some did not know what to say but wanted to communicate, so I encouraged them to ring the bells, touch her body and hold her hand. One of her grandsons came into the room and said to me, "You are doing what my Nana does. She always puts her hands on her stomach, and she said it is the only thing that helps her." It was a privilege to be present and share with Marie's family during this sacred time of her life.

For the next nine hours, I stayed with Marie, attuning her, her room and everyone in the home. The chimes outside her bedroom window continued to sound from the gentle breeze. Her outer body continued to shut down: her temperature was falling, and her breathing became more laboured. Simultaneously, I could sense the inner, more lasting planes of Marie's being were highly active and alive. Together, we moved into a timeless space of peace and bliss. I could never begin to count the number of times I used the Cosmic Symbols of TRT®, but each time I did, they seemed to merge through these different dimensions more deeply and gently. I felt I was touching beyond the gates of death to an indescribable space of love.

Her son, Danny, asked me if it would be all right to lie beside his mom. I said, "Of course," and it was so beautiful to see him there with his arm around his mom, stroking her hair and holding her hand. He prayed beside her and thanked her for being there for him throughout his life. This amazing image of mother and son, of compassion and love, will stay with me for the rest of my life. I moved my hands to Marie's feet and completed one more attunement.

It was about one in the morning, and family members found couches and chairs to fall asleep in. The house was peaceful and quiet. A night nurse was in the room next to Marie's, and Danny was sleeping beside his mom. I knew my work was over, and she was now ready. I placed a blanket over both of them and left. The night air was crisp, and as I drove away, I once again felt blessed to have TRT®, and once again, I had celebrated in this wonderful mystery of dying. I received a message on my voice mail that Marie died peacefully at six that morning. Her family's wish was for her to die peacefully, and they were so grateful for all the support.

Dynamic Inner Connection

A few days after Marie made her transition, I visited a 59-year-old man who had been diagnosed five years earlier with head and neck cancer. He was now in the end stage, and professionals were questioning what was holding him here at this point as all medical indications pointed to his death. A social worker suggested Radiant Touch® to facilitate his transition.

When I arrived, I noticed the family was exhausted. Doctors had told the family he should not be alive; it defied logic, and there he was into the 12th day, still hanging on. I had directed to him in my regular early morning session of hands-on and to myself to have no desire for outcome. 'He will go when he is ready to go, not when the doctors say and not when the family wants,' I told myself.

In the living room surrounded by his family, a picture of Jesus and all his trophies, John lay in a hospital bed in a coma. He was an avid hunter and boater and loved the outdoors. I had never met him before this day, but for the next two and a half hours, I learned a lot about him by "being" with him. In a soft voice I introduced myself and explained what I would be doing. I played a CD of nature sounds and music and began directing Attunements. I immediately gave John the Attunements for The First Degree Official Program of The Radiance Technique®, Authentic Reiki® and moved his hands to lie on his body. I placed my hands lightly on Head Positions #2, #3 and #4 and all Front Positions.

There were many shifts in his breathing over time. Such dramatic changes, I began counting his inhalations and exhalations as they moved further and further apart. This was especially noticeable on Front Positions #3 and #4. I considered the question, 'Would he go now in my hands?' I knew to be fully present, and I needed to let go of this thought. So I began again patterning Cosmic Symbols. Those thoughts left and suddenly my hands seemed to become a part of him as I gently moved them over his stomach. My hands sunk deep within him to a point that it was as if I was not in my own body, independent, but connected as one with John. I experienced swirling spirals within myself, within John and all around us. These were not physical sensations but a deep inner pulsating difficult to translate in words. I do not remember breathing or hearing John's outer breath but felt connected and supported by an inner breath that was limitless and expansive. Here was a man clearly dying on the outside, but something healing and profound was happening on the inner levels of his being. He was alive and well here.

He was dissolving and expanding at the same time. I felt joy and celebration.

His daughter came back into the room later and said that they were hoping he would die while I was there. She asked me if she should call for her children to come. She wanted to know if he was going to die very soon. I told her he would die when he was ready. I do not know what John still needed to do, but I knew within that he would not go that day. I have realized the importance of adequate pain and symptom control to keep the patient comfortable. When this happens, the inner journey has more time, and the patient experiences fewer distractions from symptoms of the physical body.

I continued to direct to John during my daily practice. Two days later, he made his transition. The existence of the continuum of the inner planes of energy was once again confirmed to me.

Inner Communication

Katherine Lenel has supported friends and students before and after they have made their transitions.

"My own experience with cancer and experiences with those who have made their transitions have helped me to see the process of life and death as a continuum which never ends," she explains. "The directing of energy to those in the process of dying, and to those who have made their transition, makes it utterly clear that although their bodies are no longer functioning, who they actually are is absolutely alive. It is just as possible to 'be with' someone no longer breathing physically as it is to be with someone physically alive. It is comforting, and very, very real.

"I saw my friend and TRT® student, Diane, a few hours before her death. She had been fighting metastatic non-Hodgkin's lymphoma for 13 years. She had studied TRT® for about six months before her death and was using it especially to help her relax and sense what was best for her to do next.

Although she was supposedly cancer-free at her death, her immune system was seriously compromised, and she was troubled by numbers of opportunistic diseases, especially attacking her lungs.

"I last saw her in the hospital on a respirator. She was naked except for a towel to cover her lower body. She was barely conscious. The machine which was helping her breathe was noisy and looked uncomfortable. I patterned Cosmic Symbols in my awareness and spoke to her. She turned her head toward my voice though her eyes were closed. I knew we were communicating. Later that night, she made her transition. I continued to direct energy to her in support of her transition. At the viewing of her body, held in a funeral home, it was so clear that she was not there in her body that I nearly laughed out loud. I sat in a pew with other mourners and directed energy to her and to the many people whose lives she touched. I experienced a great relief and release from sadness and the sense of loss."

Opening for Healing

After Barbara Koch-Donga received The Second Degree, her involvement with Hospice patients became deeper, and she found herself more relaxed. She noticed that she felt a deeper honouring for every patient, and her listening capacity had expanded to really be in the moment. She realized that every visit is precious and can be the last one.

One volunteer placement brought Barbara into the home of Mark, who was dying of lung cancer. His only caregiver was his daughter, Julie.

"When I arrived, Mark was in bed in the living room beside a window overlooking his garden. Julie was anxiously busy all around, trying to straighten out things in the room, dust and water the houseplants. I sat beside Mark's bed and began the session with Front Position #1, while directing Cosmic Symbols to Julie. I asked her to sit across from me and hold her father's hand. She did so readily. It was like she needed permission. I asked her to tell me about her father. Julie spoke quietly about how her father loved flowers and how she had learned from him about gardening. While stroking her father's hand, Julie's voice was like beautiful music, expressing love, gratitude and joy. I continued hands-on and directing and Julie stayed close by her father's side. TRT® created an opening, a healing between daughter and father. It was like a moving thank-you. Mark made his transition the next morning."

Shared Timeless Moments

Another request found Barbara in the home of Mike Murray, who had a poor prognosis of liver and colon cancer. His wish was to die at home, and his wife received a lot of help from the community but was his sole caregiver.

"My very first session of Radiant Touch® with Mike took place in his living room. Mike sat in his favourite recliner, and his wife Pauline initially sat on the couch. I began hands-on with Mike and directed Cosmic Symbols to his wife so she would receive a session as well. Mike fell asleep and so did Pauline.

"It was important that Pauline was included in this process. She shared that Mike was restless, especially in the evening. She bought a copy of the music that I used in the sessions and would begin to play it for him at night. I told her to call me and let me know what time she puts the music on. Pauline was surprised and inquired that I wouldn't come out every time, would I? I explained that I would direct to him and to her. Puzzled, I gave her a metaphor using a telephone call that she could understand. When I do hands-on, that is the local call, I said. Then when I direct Radiant energy, that is a long-distance call. This seemed to work for her.

"As Mike became weaker, it was more difficult for him to move, so the last two sessions I did with him before his death were in his bedroom. Pauline laid beside him, holding his hand and touching him gently while I did his Head and Front Positions. It was a timeless, intimate moment, and I felt deeply honoured to witness and be a part of it."

Barbara's directing energy to her clients has expanded her hospice service to others, and her metaphor of a telephone line assisted Pauline in understanding what she was doing. Unlike phone lines or emails, where sometimes you connect and sometimes get cut off, misdirected or intercepted, with TRT® you have a direct connection to Radiant transcendenal energy not dependent on outer forms or lack thereof.

Pauline writes about her experience: "I was committed to keeping Mike home and doing everything in my power to make it 'quality time.' When Hospice made sessions of TRT® available, we accepted.

"Mike was very open to receiving the sessions. No matter how much pain he was in, or how restless he was, he would relax and go off to sleep almost as soon as Barbara began the session. I would sit quietly and rest, having a break from my caregiving duties. Amazingly, I felt so relaxed and peaceful afterward, as though I, too, had received a session. Barbara explained that I did! She had directed Radiant energy to me at the same time as she gave Mike hands-on.

"Later, when Mike became weaker, he would stay in bed for his session. I wanted to just lie beside him and receive a session too. Barbara encouraged me to gently lay my hands on him as well. She gave him Radiant energy. I gave him all my love. And he would continue to sleep peacefully while Barbara and I tiptoed out of the room.

"When Mike was dying and the children and grandchildren were home, we would play the relaxation music that Barbara used, and whoever was with me would join in touching his body and just being present with our love and positive energy. Even though none of us had TRT®, being close to him was important.

"Several weeks after his death, I had the opportunity

to take The First Degree Official Program of The Radiance Technique®, Authentic Reiki®. I thought that I would be doing it just for my own benefit on my grief journey. But my Radiant hands, unbidden, began to open more and touch others.

"One time, when I was with four of my grandchildren who were all seated at the table, I stood between two of them and put my hands on their shoulders. One of the others immediately proclaimed, 'I need Grandma's hands on me!'

"As a Eucharist minister, I visit the ill at home, and one time when I brought communion to an elderly member of our parish, she complained of a headache that had lingered for a whole week. On impulse, I placed my hands on Head Position #2 and kept them there for a few minutes. She phoned me a few days later and thanked me for 'fixing' her headache.

"I attend a bereavement group since Mike's death to support me on my journey, and one night a woman sitting beside me was sharing an experience with us. I put my hand on her upper back in a gesture of comfort. She immediately said, 'Oh, please leave your hand there. That's right where I hurt and that feels so good!'

"I feel privileged and awed to have the gift of Radiant Touch® and continue to share it with others. I am looking forward to expanding into advanced degrees of The Radiance Technique® for my own unfolding journey."

Radiant Connection Beyond Words

Los Angeles Authorized Instructor, Joyce Kenyon, who has studied to The Seventh Degree, writes how she supported her father during his transition:

"My father died of metastatic prostate cancer when he was in his 80s. I have deepest gratitude that with The Radiance Technique® I was able to share his final weeks with him — easing his pain and supporting him in Radiant Light and Love.

"The cancer had spread to his liver, and he was too nauseated to eat or drink, but when I gave him attunements and hands-on, he actually sat up in bed unassisted and drank some water. Even though he was extremely thin — physically wasted — his face took on an inner glow.

"On the last day, he could not speak, but the communication between us, through my Radiant Touch®, was more eloquent than any words.

"We had always been especially close, and I feared that I would be devastated at his passing. I was amazed to find that with the universal energy of TRT®, joined with the inner planes support of my radiant friends and colleagues, I never felt a loss. Our relationship was Whole, Joyous and Complete."

Sister's Love Expands

Another Authorized Instructor and student of The Fourth Degree, Dawn Champion, shared with me the story of her sister:

"When my sister, Norma, was in her dying process, I was gifted with the opportunity to be with her. For seven days, we were connected on all levels. Before this time, I had no idea what was involved in assisting with a person's physical passing. Upon arriving in Salt Lake City, I felt the importance of this special event I was about to experience.

"Norma was at home and received visits by the hospice nurse. She was very much loved by her large family and many friends. Needless to say, there were many trying times and what seemed to be total chaos. With the steady stream of visitors and phone calls, all involved with intense emotions, feelings and fears, I was suddenly put in the role of caregiver and peacemaker. This 24 hour vigil was very demanding.

"During this process, I was living in the present, not knowing what would transpire next. With all that was happening simultaneously a beautiful, peaceful, loving Radiant energy seemed to embrace all of us and carry us as we embarked on this incredible journey into the unknown. In the natural flow of events, each member of the family had the opportunity to be alone with her and her radiant essence. While she was withdrawing from her physical existence, she maintained a sparkle in her eyes and a calm acceptance. This was a blessing to witness and behold.

"I was constantly activating and directing Radiant energy by utilizing the Advanced Degrees of TRT®. I was able to apply Radiant Touch® with Norma, myself and other members of the family often. The bonding and understanding between us was beyond words, feelings and actions. Our inner connection as sisters was brought to a new level. With TRT®, I had no feelings of helplessness. I was guided by my heart, moment to moment, on what to do.

"Many people expressed to me how much they appreciated my being there. I am the one who is thankful! I have always felt a door opens whenever someone enters or exits this world. I had a glimpse of that open gateway filled with radiant light and love where heaven and earth meet. I am deeply grateful to my sister for allowing me to share in the experience and celebration of her transition, and forever grateful for TRT®."

Students of The Radiance Technique® echo Dawn's gratitude repeatedly. This sacred energy allows us to be an escort and giver of Light to others while assisting in our own transformation at the same time.

Heart-First Devotion

Gisela Stenwald of Germany, TRT® student of The Fifth Degree, experienced her mother's rapid physical deterioration. Her mother became totally bedridden and could not even lie down. She had many orthopedic problems, most of her body was riddled with bed sores, and there was hardly any intact skin left because the ulceration was extensive and deep.

"During my regular visits to my mother in the nursing

home, I supported her with TRT® Hands-on, directing energy and attunements. What an experience for both of us. It was ever so supporting and loving; sometimes she even managed a smile, and such a smile that I will never forget. I received Radiant support from others directing to my mother and me. When her final time appeared to be near, I stayed with her continuously. It was hard to believe, with 'TRT® in action,' there was so much going on between us. There was so much closeness, love, tranquility and trust. Periodically, nurses had to drain her bronchial phlegm, and this must have been a very unpleasant procedure for her. Later, she fell into a deep sleep, and even then there was so much loving and silent communication between us. I was just around her, stroking her, doing hands-on, using Cosmic Symbols, attuning her, attuning myself and holding her feet.

"When the rattling in her bronchial tubes became more intense and prolonged, I called the nurses. They tried to free her from the accumulated phlegm but didn't succeed. I saw her sad eyes looking so helpless. The nurses laid her back on the pillow, and I saw her eyes moving upwards. I moved to put my head next to hers, talking very gently to her and knowing what was happening. Very quietly, a slight sigh came from her. While using Cosmic Symbols on the inner planes, there came a warm wave of festive stillness, love, peace and great joy, a feeling of all-pervading rapturous bliss at that moment in time.

"My mother was lying there with a tiny but relieved smile on her face, as if she was watching what was happening around her. About an hour later, my husband and daughter came up. Once everyone had gathered in the room, she died. During her moment of leaving this world, I thanked my mother for allowing me to be with her when she made her transition."

"It was as if my mother was still in this world, just listening with that little smile of hers. The three of us decided to stay with her. We did not want to leave her; we wanted to be with her. For the next six hours, I found myself talking to her, doing hands-on, caressing her. There was still so much activity inside her; it was somehow very fascinating to observe what was going on."

His Holiness the Dalai Lama explains the Buddhist view of stages after death: "According to modern science, after breathing ceases and the heart stops beating, the function of the brain stops within minutes. However, according to the Buddhist explanation, there are still another four stages to go. There are no more external indications, only internal signs or feelings. At each stage, you see different coloured lights. First whitish, then reddish, then darkness, and finally, there is a feeling of infinite space, which is known as the 'clear light.' Although the grosser levels of consciousness have ceased to exist, the subtle consciousness has not departed from the body. The ability to stay with the clear light normally belongs only to highly evolved meditators, but occasionally people become absorbed in it accidentally."[15]

Along with using TRT®, I often recommend Stephen Levine's enlightening book, *A Year to Live*. In it, he encourages everyone to commit to the experiment of living a year as though it were the last. In the practice of dying, we are able to embrace and appreciate life right here and right now. He writes, "Because we never know whether our next breath may be our last, being prepared for the immediate unknown becomes as practical as applying for a passport while still uncertain of our destination or time of departure. Without these first steps, the last steps can go badly."[16]

The cycles of life are a rich ground for exploration and self-discovery. Our medical care system continues to improve pain and symptom control, which is important. The inner journey has more time, and one is not as distracted. In the last moments, relationships are often healed, and forgiveness is accepted.

Shared Journey to the Gateway of Death

Linda Richard is an Authorized Instructor with The Seventh Degree and shares the following intimate and revealing experience:

"Several years ago I discovered that dying with joy and peace is everyone's birthright. I came to know Katherine, a beautiful woman with lung and brain cancer, through her best friend who had studied The First and Second Degree with me. Her friend asked that I give hands-on sessions to Katherine to support her. We made a connection and agreed to weekly sessions in which her friend and I joined for two-hour sessions. Katherine's emphasis was on getting well and licking the brain tumour — which she did. Though Katherine did not want to study TRT®, she wanted us to continue with these sessions to help fortify her recovery. This went on for three to four months.

"Then the news came that cancer was now evident in her lungs. It was devastating news. When I began that week's session, it seemed a soft cocoon of radiant love was holding Katherine and us. Usually loquacious, she was very quiet. I placed my hands in the positions and directed symbols throughout her being. Halfway through the session, Katherine sat up saying in a clear voice 'I am prepared to go whichever way the road turns.' I experienced such a profound love in that statement of acceptance. I always felt the Donovan song, *Love is all around us comforting. It holds you in its arms and makes your heart sing*, characterized our radiant encounters.

"Thus began our shared journey towards that great gateway we call death. I came to her home twice a week. Sometimes I was alone, and sometimes a group gathered to give hands-on. Witty Katherine had great comments, making us laugh. The group sessions filled with Radiant energy, chanting of mantras, laughter, personal stories and a delicious supper made by her husband. It was his gift to us. She saved the sad feelings for her husband's and my ears. Listening with my heart hands seemed to give me the capacity to listen and respond from my heart. Katherine came through these tough feelings with grace. She always seemed to face things directly, viewing it as part of a great adventure we call life. What I began to observe as we radiantly spent time together was that Katherine, her close friend, her husband and I were developing a discernment of what was essential to life and stripping away what was nonessential.

"As the cancer invaded her body more, she lost weight and strength, but never her wit and courage. Sometimes I would just hold her in my arms while she lay on the couch, keeping my heart hands at her heart centre or one hand at her crown and another at the heart. One day, as she lay in my arms, Katherine said, 'Linda, I need to find out what happens as you die. Can you help me?' She wanted to know if we could identify when it would occur and what happened to the physical body. So we both researched.

"Some of the symptoms indicating when the body is getting ready included: slipping down in the bed, curling into fetal positions, losing consciousness, and large evacuation of bodily fluids. Katherine planned whom she wanted with her when it occurred. She and her husband had planned the surroundings — candles, flowers, incense, special spiritual statues and pictures. I chose the music. We called it her birthday celebration, and I felt privileged to be invited.

"One night, a group of radiant people came to share hands-on with Katherine. It was a very loving, humorous evening that had a special quality of vitality to it. Katherine asked others to leave the room, as she had to go to the bathroom. She asked me to help her out of the hospital bed. I was surprised since I was not her usual partner in that aspect of caretaking. After removing the bedpan, Katherine remarked, 'Linda, I'm scudding.' Baffled, I responded, 'What do you

mean?' She said, 'Jim and I say that when we are slipping
and we did not mean to. I am scudding. Stay close.' Symbols
flooded both of us. We held hands a few moments in silence.
I nodded. We were quiet together in a heart first connection
the rest of the evening. We knew the transition was near.

"The next morning Jim called me to tell me she had lost
consciousness and was in a coma. The hospice nurse explained
how to keep her comfortable and how much time might pass.
When I arrived, her best friend and I placed our Radiant
hands on her. I started with the crown centre, attuning. I
moved to each centre, placing my hands and attuning ending at the base/security centre. Then I began spiralling up
the centres from the base again attuning each centre. We
repeated this many times throughout these hours. Her cat
came and took up residence between her legs. We had the
music, *Tibetan Bells II*, softly playing.

"For about 24 hours Katherine lay in a coma. I attuned the
other two people present, her husband and her friend. We all
embraced being with Katherine in a tender way. I did it with
TRT®, her friend with TRT® and Native American traditions,
and her husband with the years of shared loving intimacy.

"In the wee hours of the next morning, Katherine's
breathing became laboured. As the end seemed near, her husband left briefly to call her parents. At this moment, I held
her other hand. It surprised me that she gripped it harder.
Startled, I looked up at Katherine. She had a beautiful smile
and a crystal tear came from her closed eyes. I knew in that
moment that Katherine was experiencing the great LIGHT,
all that we had talked about months before — and it was OK
to pass on. I called for Jim to hurry. He returned to her side. I
was swept into the experience with her with the gift of TRT®
Cosmic Symbols. I could not think. I knew what was happening without seeing it, but it felt as though I went to the inner
plane gateway with her. Suddenly she let my hand go and she
was gone. All of us knew it at the same time.

"We sat with her for some time at peace ourselves, unable to put into words what we had experienced and were continuing to experience. After about an hour, in silence, we bathed her, anointed her body with oils and dressed her in the dress Katherine had chosen for this moment. After we hugged one another, we began the ordinary things that had to be done.

"Later her husband told me it was the most meaningful and joyous experience he had ever had. When people talked about souls remaining present for some days later, we would look at one another smiling. We knew Katherine went like a shooting star, looking ahead to her next great adventure.

"I came to know her mother after Katherine's transition. She also had similar wit and wisdom. She was known by the nickname *Magic*, which suited her. Her husband died a year later. Magic said, 'My God, we do know how to die!' Yes, I discovered that dying in peace and joy is everyone's birthright. It is their choice. Death from our mortal body is meant to be embraced and nurtured. It is an important stage of our lives. It does not have to be a horrible time.

"Yes, there is loss of beloved ones, and we who are left are very sad. And yet, never before had I experienced such aliveness, joy, heart first connection and love in such an intimate relationship with someone dying. It was the powerful embrace of The Radiance Technique®, which held us while allowing us to have the experiences of what was *real*. I was liberated from our cultural perceptions of tragedy, 'such a shame, the grim reaper come to cut you down in the prime of life.' Instead, when accepted and faced directly, there is so much support — both on inner and outer planes. It is a glorious dance. One is preparing to move from form to formless and love is all that matters. People who came to visit Katherine would remark in wonderment how they came to cheer her, but somehow she cheered them.

"The following are two insights I had from his amazing experience:

- After being with Katherine in this extraordinary journey, I expected everyone else's dying to be like that. It was not so. I realized that it was related to each person's consciousness. My father never wanted to look at what would be beyond this life. So his passing was a different experience.

- I have found that it is best to let the Radiant cosmic energy in TRT®lead me when I am with someone. I do not impose myself into the process. I place my hands in the positions taught to us, generate Cosmic Symbols and attunements. Then I let the energy carry us, spiralling into the unknown. It leads the recipient to open up to what they need to talk about and/or process. It also leads me to say what needs to be said."

Linda's testimonial along with others in this chapter illustrate one of TRT®'s deeper inner aspects:

The Radiance Technique® and its direct access to Radiant, Light-energy allows for contact with all levels of the person's Being and provides a safe, natural technique for supporting the releasing of energy from the body at death. ...[17]

[1] Ray, *The Expanded Reference Manual of The Radiance Technique®, Authentic Reiki®*, p. 29.

[2] Jane Buckle, R.N., *Clinical Aromatherapy in Nursing*, (London, England: Arnold Publishing, 1997), p. 229.

[3] Gelek Rimpoche, Ann Arbor Jewel Heart *Odyssey to Living Summer Retreat* 2002, Michigan, USA.

[4] Ray, *The Expanded Reference Manual of The Radiance Technique®, Authentic Reiki®*, p. 37.

[5] Ganga Stone, *Start the Conversation*, (New York, NY: Warner Books, Inc., 1996), p. 22.

[6] Richard Gerber, MD. *A Practical Guide to Vibrational Medicine*, (New York, NY: HarperCollins, 2000), p. 12.

[7] Gehlek Nawang Rimpoche, *Good Life, Good Death: Tibetan Wisdom on Reincarnation*, (New York, NY: Riverhead Books, 2001). p. 31.

[8] Sogyal Rinpoche, *The Tibetan Book of Living and Dying*, (New York, NY: HarperCollins, 1994), p. 259.

[9] Ray, *The Expanded Reference Manual of The Radiance Technique®, Authentic Reiki®*, p. 23.

[10] Peter Knudtson & David Suzuki, *Wisdom of the Elders*, (Toronto, ON: Stoddart Publishing Co. Ltd., 1992), p. 41.

[11] *The Bible*, King James Version Ecclesiasties 12: 6.

[12] Gehlek Nawang Rimpoche, *Good Life, Good Death*, p. 33.

[13] Sogyal Rinpoche, *The Tibetan Book of Living and Dying*, p. 256.

[14] Barbara Ray, Ph.D., *The 'Reiki' Factor in The Radiance Technique®*, (St. Petersburg, FL: Radiance Associates, 1992), p. 97.

[15] His Holiness the Dalai Lama, *The Joy of Living and Dying*, (New York, NY: The Library of Tibet Inc., HarperCollins, 1997), p. 44.

[16] Stephen Levine, *A Year to Live*, (New York, NY: Bell Tower, 1997), p. 13.

[17] Ray, *The 'Reiki' Factor in The Radiance Technique®, Authentic Reiki®*, p. 101.

The Light of God before me.
The Light of God behind me.
The Light of God above me.
The Light of God beside me.
The Light of God within me.

~ from The Prayer of St. Patrick

Transforming Grief

Even with medication prescribed by my family doctor to help me with depression and lack of sleep due to the stress of my wife's illness and death, I was mentally fatigued, disoriented and physically exhausted. I truly believe that had it not been for The Radiance Technique®, I would probably have suffered a stroke or heart attack and am not sure of the quality of life that I would have had.

I do believe The Radiance Technique® saved my life.

~ Caregiver Evaluation

-8-

HOW WE CONSCIOUSLY FEEL ABOUT THE CYCLE of death is directly related to how we handle our journey of grief and sorrow. How we understand dying — an ending, a beginning or a continuation — affects how we deal with transition. We touch into the depths of our souls. Our perceived loss on the outer creates many physical, emotional and psychological changes. Often, this moment is a time of reflection and evaluation. It can also be a time of celebration. The previous chapter was filled with many experiences of people documenting the dynamic interaction of the more inner and subtle energy shifts before, during and after death of the physical body. And just as each experience was unique, the way in which we grieve is as individual as our thumb print. No way is right and no way is wrong, but there are some experiences that are common to all. "When we are in grief, our eyes are blurred, our ears are plugged, our throat constricted unable to speak, and our inner stomach is tight,"[1] relates Professor Castenda, a Mohawk elder.

Emotions and the organs of the body are interrelated, and there is a direct relationship of how the body reacts to the stress of sadness. When I was diagnosed with cancer, I learned a lot about my physical and emotional body through Kate Kent, Dipl.Ac., C.H., my acupuncturist. In TCM (Traditional Chinese Medicine), the meridian lines have no correspondence to the anatomical map that we have. According to Kate, "The emotion of sadness weakens the Lung Qi, which can be felt in the pulse of someone going through a trauma.

In Chinese medicine theory, the lungs govern Qi, and if this is depleted, it will lead to exhaustion, depression, crying, hopeless and helpless feelings and breathlessness."[2]
· Such intense emotional losses contribute to a lowered immune system, and the effects of bereavement on surviving spouses are documented. The Cancer Project of the Physicians Committee for Responsible Medicine writes about one study published in Lancet: "In a landmark study, R.W. Bathrop, M.D., and his colleagues at the University of New South Wales in Sydney, Australia, studied the effects of bereavement by following the lives of surviving spouses and charting changes in immune function during mourning. At eight weeks, T-cell functions were significantly lower in the bereaved spouses than in age-and-sex-matched controls."[3]

I came to know and experience that the energy of The Radiance Technique® is supportive for restoring depleted energy to the whole body and connecting to feelings that surface during grief and bereavement.

Grief, Grieving — ... *The Radiance Technique® can be used to access whole energy that is supportive to a natural unfolding of the feelings that can accompany the grieving process. Spending time daily to apply the entire hands-on session gives you the opportunity to be with yourself and explore your feelings, releasing them in ways that are safe and harmless to yourself....* [4]

When caring for a loved one is over, it is normal to feel both grieved and relieved. As we covered in the chapter *Caregivers Along the Way*, a caregiver needs time to refuel, and when their caring ends, time seems like all they have, and in these moments, deep emotions and feelings surface.

The Role of Belief and Cultural Heritage

Religious belief, culture and family traditions also play a vital role in an individual's experience of grief. It is important to have an awareness of the various perceptions, attitudes and beliefs surrounding death and mourning. In practicing or receiving The Radiance Technique®, no religion, dogma or doctrine is involved, except whatever the practitioner or receiver chooses to bring to it. Over the years, I have supported many people from many religious faiths. People want the best care for their loved one and a peaceful transition. I have often followed pastoral care after a patient has received their last rites supporting the patient in their passage. Helping families cope includes having respect for their beliefs and cultural heritage. Participating in funerals, memorials, wakes, special ceremonies and rituals helps families grieve, as well as the people involved in caregiving. Being there to provide support in the first week, the first month and the first year can be very healing. People leave an imprint on us, on our lives. In the grieving process, TRT® plays a nurturing role helping to find unexpected sources of strength.

Healing Grief and Nurturing Self

The following story illustrates the physical and emotional connections of grief by Christa Papineau, who began her bereavement journey through the transition of her husband.

"Fear, despair, anger and isolation were among the mountain of feelings I experienced in the weeks and months following my husband's death. Robert died of leukemia after only being diagnosed for two weeks. At age thirty-three, he was otherwise a healthy man who took care of myself and our son, Adrian, who was three and a half.

"I found myself wanting to reach out to anything to stop the pain, to make everything all right again. It was beginning to be more and more difficult to put on the happy face everyone was accustomed to seeing.

"I received a phone call from a hospice social worker offering many of their services, and she recommended a series of sessions of The Radiance Technique® in conjunction with counselling. I had heard of this before, when my cousin was losing her husband to cancer, and she found this was the only thing that relieved many of the symptoms of this disease. I also was told during a casual conversation with a friend how she attended a few TRT® sessions, and it helped her dramatically by reducing the pain she felt in her shoulder as a result of a past injury.

"I was always skeptical in trying non-conventional means of therapy, but out of an inner interest, I decided to give it a try. Along with the emotional pain, I also suffered from physical pain caused by fibromyalgia that was triggered from a head-on collision a year prior. I was constantly on an up-and-down roller coaster trying to handle the flare-ups. I didn't know that what I was going to experience would change the quality of my life and, by doing this, enhance the lives of those around me.

"After the first session, I experienced a deeply relaxed state that I have never experienced before. During the following weeks and sessions, I found that many of my pessimistic thoughts about my life were changing into optimistic thoughts, and I had this inner serenity that I could not explain. I also noticed that the severity of my pain had diminished, and my sleeping habits were greatly improving. How was this happening? I began to ask Christine (the person who was applying TRT®) many of my questions, and she offered a course where I could learn how to do TRT® on myself and others. I immediately knew I had to attend.

"During the course, I learned about the various chakras and the way the energy of TRT® works to bring about the highest good. At times, I felt a huge rush of energy, while at other times tears filled my eyes, and a release of tension in my chest. The most dramatic part I discovered was my sense of lightness. This feeling continued throughout my day, and often others would comment on the good spirit I was in. I felt it physically relieve tension and stiffness as well as emotionally free me from obsessions that would drag me down and steal my attention away from the important things.

"I would have to leave my son in the care of others during my classes and appointments several times throughout the day. I would usually have a strong feeling of guilt, along with a nagging depression that would often make me rush through my activities in order to return to him as quickly as possible. After my first few sessions of TRT®, that feeling of guilt lessened, and I was able to enjoy my outings with the self-confidence that I was taking care of myself. I know that applying The Radiance Technique® to myself and others has greatly improved my self-worth and connection with others.

"I often experienced much anxiety while driving in heavy traffic, mostly due to my car accident. I found that by supporting myself with Front Position #4, a sense of wellness and protection eased my nervousness to the point that I found I was able to travel to areas that I would have frequently avoided in the past.

"I start my day with a twenty minute session, completing all Head Positions. I find that my mind is clear and alert; I feel self-confident and a sense of openness towards the day ahead. Most often in the evening, I will complete the session with the Front and Back Positions. This is an essential part of relaxing my muscles and relieving tension that may have built up from the day's events. I find that I am able to let go of any fears and stress and quiet my mind from recreating the day's events. I have a feeling of gratitude for the day, and feel calm and serene. The fact that I am actively taking time to nurture myself is one of the vital acts necessary for self-love."

Expanding Dimensions of Being

Frequently, many people ask, "Don't you find this area of work hard to do and difficult?" The way I answer is that I know hospice care could be less life-giving and more draining and fatiguing emotionally and physically if I did not have a tool like TRT® to support myself and others.

It seems appropriate to share the following excerpt from a letter that was read and distributed to all family and friends at Van Ault's memorial service in May of 1996. Van was an influential mentor for me and supported me in deepening my study of TRT®, becoming a TRT® Authorized Instructor and writing this book. When this letter was read, I experienced (in my outer bodies) what the Mohawk elder related in the beginning of this chapter. Simultaneously, I had a deep celebration. Van was now free of the pain and suffering from his AIDS-related symptoms, and just as he was at his moment of death, he will always be with me.

As you say your last good-byes to me, I want to let you know that though you cannot see me, I will always be with you. The connections we have made with each other in this life speak of a deeper link, and from that link, you and I will forever be friends. Physical embodiment is only one part of the Whole experience. We can be together anytime, any place, through that place of lovely peace and quiet within us. Go there, and if you call me, I will be, also. Think of this not as the end of our relationship, but simply a shift in the form![5]

After Van's death, and right up through today, I continue to direct and inner connect with him. Many of my clients who live through a loved one's "death" speak of interesting experiences. Some share that they feel the presence of their spouse around them; others actually converse and get feedback, while still others have shared of unusual things happening like lights and fans mysteriously going on and off. These sharings often begin with, "I don't want you to think I am crazy but..."

I find that Ganga Stone's new method of grief management resonates with seeing life as a continuum. She directs others to envision the person who died as being simply out of town for the moment, knowing that they are alive somewhere. I can understand how this can help the mind. It is a start. TRT® provides the opportunity to give you direct contact and experience from the energy of the whole. So, we all start where we are, and we have an amazing possibility to embrace so much more than we think. With all this in my heart I, too, question the permanence of grief and wonder if it is more about change and sadness. Dr. Barbara Ray has the following wisdom to share which I found very helpful on the topic of continuum:

> *Continuum — An uninterrupted, <u>non-fragmented</u>, whole <u>succession</u>, interrelated and interconnected; that which is endless, continuous, unbroken, everlasting. The Radiance Technique® accesses these qualities — everlasting and enduring. As you apply The Radiance Technique®, you are supporting your unfolding process and expanding your capacities to become aware of your Real Inner Life and the continuum in all life forms — yourself, others, trees, plants, animals, the clouds, the mountains, the rivers.[6]*

I began to recognize how many little "deaths" I have experienced and that I have grieved throughout my lifetime in transitions of jobs, schools, relocations, changes in physical capacities, separations, and divorce, while including the loss of family members and clients with whom I have shared my life. I began to realize that I mourn the aspects of my life that changed. "Loss creates a barren present, as if one were sailing on a vast sea of nothingness. Those who suffer loss live suspended between a past for which they long and a future for which they hope,"[7] says Alan Wolfelt, Ph.D., Director of the Centre for Loss and Life Transition in Fort Collins, CO.

TRT® supports past, present and future. Anticipatory

grief involves past, present and future loss experiences. I found it very helpful to read about these different levels and put a name to what I have experienced over and over again. According to Chris Byrne, M.Ed., grief and bereavement specialist, "Grief during illness is stimulated by losses that have already occurred in the past, those that are currently occurring as well as those losses yet to come:

Past:
> Grief for health of person lost to disease.
> Grief for altered relationship to person and lifestyle as the result of illness.

Present:
> Grief as you witness the on-going deterioration of a person, increasing dependency, continual uncertainty, decreasing control; mourning what is gradually slipping away right now.

Future:
> Grief for plans that will never be realized in future; loneliness, social discomfort, insecurity, lifestyle changes, and changes in family roles.
> This anticipatory grief occurs on three levels:
> 1. Within the self as an individual.
> 2. Between self and dying person.
> 3. Between self and family members."[8]

A Husband's Grief

An example of past, present and future loss is illustrated through a recent client who was a caregiver. I remember receiving an urgent call from a nurse at The Ford Motor Company who had a worker on the line that had collapsed, and they did not know what to do with him. He recently lost his wife to cancer and was not coping well. His biggest problem was that he was not sleeping at all. As soon as his head hit the pillow, he was wide awake. His employers were concerned for his safety and for others. I scheduled an appointment for Ken that same evening.

Ken was a welder and described himself as a mental wreck as he continually felt that there was something more he could have done to change what happened to his wife. During our first session, I just let him talk, vent his concerns, his anger and his grief, the whole time of two hours directing TRT® to support him on the inner and outer planes. Physically, he relaxed into the chair, his face softened and his tone changed, and he commented on how much better he felt.

For the following day's session, while Ken was lying on the table, he shared that he experienced a deep feeling of relaxation and calm throughout his body and mind that he had not reached before. The next few sessions brought a deeper connection to his emotions and allowed him to release. Ken described his hands-on sessions as . For the first time, he felt an inner peace he could not describe.

A month and a half later, Ken was sleeping better, had more energy, experienced emotional pain relief and felt an increase in his ability to cope with the loss of his wife. He felt the sessions allowed time for his own personal healing, and he realized he did not need to always keep busy and be full of stress. We talked about ways he could reduce the stress in his life and be gentle with his self. I referred Ken for bereavement counselling for on-going support. On his final evaluation, Ken wrote, "Even with medication prescribed by my family doctor to help me with depression and lack of sleep due to the stress of my wife's illness and death, I was mentally fatigued, disoriented and physically exhausted. I truly believe that had it not been for The Radiance Technique®, I would probably have suffered a stroke or heart attack and am not sure of the quality of life that I would have had. I do believe The Radiance Technique® saved my life."

A few months later, Ken enrolled in training to learn The First Degree Official Program of The Radiance Techique®, Authentic Reiki®. The hands-on support has carried him to a place beyond coping, to a place of acceptance and healing. Getting to this place of acceptance takes time, and moving through the pain instead of staying in it demonstrates a deeper understanding that the experience is part of a greater whole.

Moving Through Feelings

Barbara Koch-Donga, a Hospice volunteer, explains how TRT® carried her after her son's death and helped her heal.

"After my son, Matthias, died in a car accident at the age of twenty, Hospice offered me counselling support and TRT®. I had done yoga and meditation exercises, but the sessions of Radiant Touch® had a different quality. TRT® combined with counselling allowed me to explore more deeply my inner feelings and move through them. Looking back now, I experienced the hour at each session as an island I was resting on before I had to swim further. I lived fully during that hour, accepted everything. I experienced my grief and sadness like black veils hanging over me, like black clouds passing over me. I had this image of swimming through a deep black lake, and all I remember was Christine saying, 'As long as you keep swimming.'

"I received The First Degree in May 1997. Practising TRT® on myself was, for me, like escaping a whirlpool of thoughts, emotions and painful memories. I had also experienced intense pain in my diaphragm and rib area. I used to wake up every Saturday night at the time my son had been killed, and I was not able to go back to sleep. There was nothing I wanted to do because everything felt so senseless. The gentle touch of TRT® carried me through those hours and helped with the pain. I used all twelve positions for as long as I was awake.

"During working hours, grief would come over me like waves, and I often went to a quiet place to just do the Head Positions. These positions released my tears and calmed me down.

"It was like my son's death prepared me for my mother's death which happened a year later. I flew to Germany for my mother's funeral. I laid in my mother's bed with all her scents around me. Placing my hands on myself, TRT® released my tears. The position which comforted me the most was when I laid on my right side with my arms crossed over my heart and my left hand resting under my cheek. While in this self embrace, I remembered a line of a German poem, *Deine Hand unter meine Wange gelegt, und ich kann schlafen. (Your hand lies under my cheek, and I can sleep.)*

Barbara's experiences through grieving led her to volunteering. In her cycle of healing, she began assisting others in their transition as she movingly shared in the previous chapter. She continues here with another powerful experience during the final hours of a patient named Susan, "In her restlessness and feeling her family's pain, Susan asked me to help her die. So, during hands-on, I shared with her a story of my mother. I told her that during one of my last visits, my mother and I travelled together to the province of Friesland. While there, I saw high in the sky, the first double rainbow in my life. It became a link between my mother and me. My mother's death notice included a quote from my mother, She had wanted to die, and she used to say, On the top of the notice, my brothers and sisters chose a picture of a double rainbow. I shared with Susan that I could walk with her up to the bridge, but that she would have to cross it by herself. I also told her I would ask my mother to wait for her on the other side, to be there for her. She felt comforted and slowly closed her eyes again. She was able to relax deeply and fell asleep.

"The day after Susan's death, I was driving into Windsor. The sun was rising in the east, and dark clouds were looming in the northwest. It started to rain. I was thinking about Susan, and suddenly there was a huge rainbow like a portal to the sky spanning the horizon. As I continued to look, I saw there was a second rainbow closer to the sunrise. A double rainbow.

"The rainbow is my link to my mother, and since she died, a link to the other dimension. It shows me that we need the sun and the rain to create this, and it can come and disappear in seconds. The rainbow reminded me of how precious life is. It let me realize how fortunate I am to be able to touch and hold people in Radiant Light. With every one of them whom I touched, I connected as if I wove a fine thread to their hearts, and if I keep doing it, I will be able to create a web of wonderful feelings. I realize that I connect to this transcendental energy which sets my hands on fire, makes my legs shake and gives the receiver a wonderful gift. So, after all, I have found a place for all this leftover love I feel for my dead son and dead mother."

One Breath at a Time

No one expects their child to die before them. Barbara's personal experience with her son enabled her to help fellow volunteer Pat Bachand. The nurturing energy of TRT® continues to sustain Pat after the death of her daughter.

"On December 11, 2003, our family experienced a most painful lesson of life," she explains. "Our 37-year-old daughter Andrea made her transition as a result of a blood clot. A simple car accident landed her in the hospital for a surgery on her foot. This seemed all so simple on the outer, but on the inner I felt something was terribly wrong. They said it was the trauma, medication and stress.

"The ambulance left our house at 9:50 am. I picked up

my husband at work. I told him Andrea just needed different medication. Thank God my husband Brian came with me. By noon it was over. Our beautiful daughter had made her transition.

"The pain is beyond words! I thank God every day for TRT®.

"A mother cradles her child within her womb. Then on the glorious day of birth when Andrea was placed in my arms, I felt like I had the whole world in my arms. Our child, a precious gift.

"We held her, loved her and watched her grow and become the beautiful, radiant person she was. On that day in the cold of December, I cradled my child for the last time in this physical world. I sat and gently held Andrea's head for a very long time, even after she died.

"We are blessed with a very loving group of family, friends and TRT® friends, all of whom have given us great love, support and strength. They are our light on this long dark road we travel.

"The pain is always present. TRT® is a tool to see the pain walk with me, beside me, but I am not allowing the pain to consume me. My daily hands-on sessions and receiving Radiant energy from our friends around the globe has also allowed me to see the gifts Andrea still continues to send. Giving myself sessions is a gift, my blanket of comfort. It provides me with deep peace and acceptance of each unfolding moment. I feel my inner and outer planes coming to balance, allowing me to be fully present with each moment, each breath. A day at a time but very often a breath at a time, and I am radiantly supported going into the next breath. "

Both Pat and Barbara's journey in grieving, like many, reveals that grief has no time limits or schedule and is something mysterious to be honoured. In families, the pressure is to get on with your life, that somehow talking about loved ones, about our feelings brings the aspect of death too close for comfort. It is like the story about the elephant in the room. In the middle of the room stands an elephant, and everyone is talking over, under and around the elephant but never acknowledging that the elephant is in the room. If we are to mourn our grief and heal ourselves, we need to be able to express our feelings and recognize time is needed.

Release of Multiple Losses

Multiple deaths in a short period of time are difficult, as Hospice volunteer Gloria Smith discovered:

"Annie was 71 when she lost both her husband and her 38-year-old daughter five months apart. Her daughter was actively being treated for cancer at the time of her husband's death, and Annie held in her grief so she could be supportive of her daughter's treatment and well-being. Our first session together was a few weeks after her daughter's death.

"Within twenty minutes of our first Radiant Touch® session, during Head Position #4, Annie started to cry deeply and did so for the remainder of the hour. I connected to this pain, and I also started to cry very softly. As I continued the session, I felt both her and I were in an expansive ocean of loss. Yet, somehow, within this loss, I felt immense calm and loving Radiant energy supporting us within and without in healing and comfort. At the end of the session, Annie shared with me she felt immense healing around her heart area and on the left side of her body. She was being treated for attacks of partial paralysis when she would tighten up which had manifested after her daughter's death. She felt lighter and a great release from the grief she had been holding since the death of her husband. I was very moved by the love and healing of TRT®. I am very grateful for the growth and healing I have experienced as a result of my continued daily use of The Radiance Technique® and my expansion into The Radiant Third Degree."

Letting Go

A young woman was referred to me by a social worker because she was having a particularly difficult time grieving for her husband. It had been eight months since his death, and Karen had not cried or expressed her emotions. She grew up in a family that was particularly forceful in the fact that you don't show your feelings and just learn to move on. Karen had individual counselling and attended a support group but still felt detached from her real self. This way of coping might have served her in the past, but it certainly was not supporting her now, she concluded. Karen expressed to me that she did feel empty and felt there was no peace in her life.

Karen's first session of TRT® connected her to inner levels she had cut off. As she relaxed in a safe and quiet space, the layers of outer energy she had used for protection began to peel away. By the time I reached Front Position #1, a few tears began to roll down her cheeks, and then she began to sob deeply and loudly. For the remainder of the session, I always kept my left hand on her heart centre and moved my right hand to complete the Front Positions. I also spent extra time on Front Position #3 because Karen expressed that she had a lot of pain there. I knew from experience as well that this position, the solar plexus chakra, assists in the need for control on all levels. Karen summed up her experiences in an evaluation: "The inner feelings of grief came out like an explosion. I see things and people around me differently. The inner peace I can now achieve was realized at my Radiant Touch® sessions."

Some say that our body becomes calloused by frequent grief if we let it. I remember a patient in a support group at Hospice questioning, For patients and caregivers in a Hospice support group, loss and death of fellow members becomes a part of it. At this particular time, there were quite a few deaths that had happened close together. Some members left the group and said that they had to leave to see that there is life out there. It is true we often hear what loss has taken from us, so it becomes appropriate to celebrate what the dying person has given us. It is from this focus that the group was able to continue on together.

Blessed are they who mourn for they will be comforted.[9]

Hospice nurses, social workers, support staff and volunteers are faced with multiple deaths in a short period of time. When people all around you are dying, it can be difficult. As discussed earlier, how we mourn is related to our consciousness about what happens to a person when they die. In any case, it is important to set time as an individual as well as a group to honour and acknowledge a person's transition. It can be a time for coming together to comfort one another.

During special support nights for Radiant Touch® volunteers, we take time in the beginning of our evening to create a circle to acknowledge the people we are all supporting as well as those who have made their transition. Time is created to share special memories or gifts we have received from the experience of connecting to the life of another human being. Simply, it provides a time for contemplation within ourselves to honour timeless moments we have shared.

When we are sad, we begin to search for meaning as we feel we enter the wilderness of our soul. We try to find meaning in all of this suffering. This time of contemplation and turning inward requires a lot of gentleness towards us. As Christa Papineau observed, "The fact that I am actively taking time to nurture myself is one of the vital acts necessary for self-love."

Dealing with changes in our relationships is challenging. You never forget, but in time, you do transition to a space within that is less painful. What follows are some suggestions for radiantly supporting yourself in your grieving process.

Getting the Help You Need
Suggestions for Supporting Your Grieving Process

- **Connect to your body**
  Begin walking or start a gentle exercise program after you have seen your doctor. Some gentle movement like beginner's hatha yoga or tai chi. Be open to touch like therapeutic massage, reflexology or aromatherapy to assist in "feeling" yourself again.

- **Nourish your body**
  Try to eat regular meals. Warm foods like soup are very comforting at this time. Seek advice of a qualified health care practitioner regarding vitamin/mineral/herbal supplements. If you find you don't want to cook, go out for dinner, let friends invite you or seek support from a local Meals-on-Wheels community program.

- **Nourish your spiritual self**
  Special spiritual texts that have meaning to you can be a comfort and support as well as prayers or songs of healing.

- **Connect to nature**
  Observe the cycles and rhythms around you. Be present to the moment and gifts the natural world can share with you. Natural sounds in nature are also healing.

- **Seek support**
  If it feels right for you, seek support of a bereavement counsellor or support group. Let friends support you, and at the same time, be honest if you need time alone.

  Request your name be included on The Radiant TRT Heart First Ashram® Healing/Wholing Network of The Radiance Technique International Association, Inc., for receiving directing of Radiant energy support.

- **Support your "whole" self**
  With hands-on sessions of TRT® at least twice a day, giving special emphasis for nurturing on Head Position #3 and Front Position #1. The nourishing and meditative aspects of TRT® support your unfolding journey.

  Receive sessions from local Radiant Touch® practitioners and friends who have studied TRT®. You might even ask for a Radiant Touch® marathon.

- **Remembering is healing**
  Active remembering and cherishing is healing. The memories can be like food for your soul — creating a soulful connection in ordinary places you walk, pictures you look at, friends and family you visit.

- **Celebrate special moments**
  Create special moments for remembering and continuing your relationship of your loved one. Recognize their value by celebrating how events and people have shaped your life. Many cultures have specific ceremonies to mark beginnings, endings and honouring those who have passed before us. You can create your own ceremony, whether it is reciting a prayer, planting a tree, lighting a fire or preparing a meal. It can be anything that is meaningful to you. You can do it yourself or involve others. Establishing rituals are effective bereavement tools in coping with change.

  You may also consider having a memorial service sometime after the funeral. It could be a month later, or even a year later. It is a time to come together to comfort one another in community. It is a time for celebrating life legacies and special moments. You could make it an annual event and invite family and friends.

- **Direct Radiant Energy**
  Students of TRT® who have studied The Second Degree have learned a precise method for directing Radiant Energy beyond time and space. You may direct energy to a special time that you had spent with your loved one. You may also direct to your loved one's forever self in

the here and now.
- **Be gentle with yourself**
Honour the changes you feel. Give yourself time to heal.

[1] Professor Castenda, Mohawk Elder, Speech at 1999 Conference on Care for the Terminally Ill, Montreal, Quebec.

[2] Kate Kent, Dipl. Ac., C.H. (NCCAOM)Dr. Ac. Article in *Vitality* magazine October 1994 "Grieving — Chinese Medicine for Emotional Pain," p. 22.

[3] The Cancer Project, 5100 Wisconsin Ave., NW, Suite 400, Washington, DC, http://www.cancerproject.org/survival/cancer_facts/exercise.php

[4] Barbara Ray, Ph.D., *The Expanded Reference Manual of The Radiance Technique*®, *Authentic Reiki*®,(St. Petersburg, FL: Radiance Associates, 1987), p. 46.

[5] Van R. Ault, *An Open Letter to All My Friends*, drafted July 1992.

[6] Ray, *The Expanded Reference Manual of The Radiance Technique*®, *Authentic Reiki*®, p. 24.

[7] Alan Wolfelt, "Caring for Ourselves as We Care for Others Conference," May 2000, Windsor, Ontario.

[8] Excerpted from The Hospice of Windsor & Essex County Inc. Volunteer Training Manual, Chapter Grief and Bereavement, C. Byrne, 2001.

[9] *The Bible*, King James Version, Matthew 5: 4.

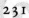

PART 5

Receiving the gift to
Access the
Divine
I nner planes in
Abundance of healing and
Never ending love
Celebrating our
E ternal life.

~ Patricia Bachand

Exploring TRT® with Other Modalities

When I work with clients, I always begin with one hand over their solar plexus and the other over their forehead and do inner Attunements. Within a few minutes, an inner connection, an inner communication is established, even on the very first visit. This state of relaxation and trust could never be possible in such a short time without the nurturing supportive energy of TRT®.

~ Miki Ivancsics
Shiatsu Practitioner
Authorized Instructor of The Radiance Technique®

9

THE RADIANCE TECHNIQUE® IS A WONDERFUL stand-alone therapy or can be combined with other modalities. In this chapter, we will explore a variety of modalities that have been used with others to support their process and in creating a healing environment. The suggestions in this chapter complement a TRT® session and might serve as a catalyst for comfort and pleasure and contribute to enhancing a person's perceived quality of life.

Although there are many complementary therapies, only a few are discussed here for illustration. Long time practitioners of TRT® have discovered the most important healing environment is their inner environment. This inner point of stillness and peace comes from within one's being and radiates out in every gesture of touch, word and silent presence.

Radiant Touch® and Massage

We all know how great a back rub feels, and the healing touch of massage in combination with TRT® is a wonderful experience. Our skin contains many thousands of small nerve fibres, and application of massage assists in many health benefits that affect the nervous, endocrine and circulatory system. I have used massage as well as The 'M' Technique® with referrals to my private practice. My rhythm is slower than most practitioners, as I incorporate various hands-on positions in my massage treatment that facilitate a deeper and quicker relaxing of the muscular, respiratory and nervous systems. As well, my clients have told me that release of physical pain happens quicker and this relief lasts longer. Many massage therapists receive these same comments after they have taken training in TRT®. A different quality to their massage and massage routine ensues.

Using Cosmic Symbols and attunements before and during the session also promotes a healing environment and allows me to remain focused on the healing session. They also support me in not feeling fatigued. Mixing and creating blends of oils provide another opportunity to use my hands to connect with the life force within the botanicals.

At the beginning, if the client is able to lie on his/her stomach, I begin with hands-on Head Positions #2 and #3, then move to Back Positions #1 and #3, and hold these positions for a few minutes each while I simultaneously use Cosmic Symbols. This gentle beginning helps the client to move more fully into the experience and let his/her cares of the day float away. Sometimes I will outwardly pattern Cosmic Symbols on parts of the body that seem to call for extra attention and light energy.

For clients who are unable to lie flat, I will do gentle massage to the face, head and hands while they are sitting. I use this opportunity to spend more time in the Head Positions to support the process.

Miki Ivancsics has a busy practice in Vienna, Austria, as a Shiatsu Practitioner and Authorized Instructor of TRT®. She has studied to The Sixth Degree of TRT® and describes her approach and its results:

"I am a Licensed Shiatsu Practitioner trained in a variety of traditional Thai and Taoist massage techniques that support the well-being and harmony of the outer planes -physical, mental and emotional.

"I combine different exercises for myself with the use of TRT®. One hour hands-on with inner attunements is the absolute daily minimum of what I need for myself. From there I try to stay connected with my inner body while I am practising different exercises for my body like yoga, Japanese meridian stretches, the Five Tibetans and others according to my needs, which vary from day to day. During these exercises, I combine breathing with Radiant Cosmic Symbols. Using The Radiance Technique® helped me to experience quite quickly the essence, the inner meaning of different kinds of exercises and techniques. It feels like having an inner teacher inside of me, telling me exactly what to do to exercise more precisely and effectively.

"My outer planes are on a journey too; they constantly have to expand and stretch with me and so does my exercise schedule. The purpose of my exercises is to balance my outer planes so they can serve more easily the inner planes. Through my daily TRT® meditation, I *know* from inside when it is time to adjust again.

"When I work with clients, I always begin with one hand over their solar plexus and the other over their forehead and do inner attunements. Within a few minutes, an inner connection, an inner communication is established, even on the very first visit. This state of relaxation and trust could never be possible in such a short time without the nurturing and supportive energy of TRT®.

"From this inner contact, I let myself be guided from my hands and my intuition into a session of body work. After learning different kinds of massage techniques separately and exercises separately, I now combine them according to what the client needs and is willing and able to experience and explore from within. TRT® seems to stretch the time, so that I can do more and it expands the capacity of the client to receive. I always attune the session to support wholeness and harmony.

"Through my own continuous journey and ongoing process, I have gained more insights and I am ever unfolding into compassion, acceptance and understanding for myself and for the processes, diseases and difficulties clients are experiencing, not necessarily with the mind, but with the inner heart, allowing it to be whatever is in this moment. When I am able to be an inner-non-judging-loving observer, my Radiant hands *see* and *feel* the pain inside of clients and radiate through it. I am part of this process, and I am always honoured, touched and impressed by the gentle power of the healing/wholing energy accessed by TRT®. My Radiant hands know when to stop and just be there at a certain area and when to move on.

"Using The Radiance Technique® co-creates an expanded energy field in which the client can take the opportunity to initiate self-healing and/or allow stimulation for healing and wholing. TRT® enhances the fullness and wholeness of the specific treatments I am doing."

Reflexology

My first introduction to reflexology was in 1986, when I attended an introductory foot course at a local college. From that moment, I just loved reflexology. I was amazed to learn that directly under our feet are over seven thousand nerve endings, and throughout our entire body are thousands of reflex points located not only on our feet, but also on our hands, head, and ears.

I used reflexology in my healing journey and later took a certification course to be a reflexologist. Its history, like many healing arts, is ancient. One can even view Egyptian petrographs of foot reflexology taking place. After I studied The First Degree Official Program of The Radiance Technique®, Authentic Reiki®, I learned to combine the two modalities together. It's such a natural combination, in fact, at no time when I am touching a person's feet am I not connecting with the Radiant energy within them. Over the years I have gone deep into the subtle energies of the reflex points and utilized the Cosmic Symbols at these points. People are moved into a relaxed state much more quickly than normal. I have especially found this to be true when working on ear reflex points.

Kate Goulden, a Complementary Therapist in a Devon Hospice, also has combined reflexology with TRT®, both personally and professionally:

"Working with reflexology and relaxation therapy with people facing death, I am aware of a different quality and depth in the energy levels when patterning the Cosmic Symbols. When I work on the spinal reflexes in micro-spirals from the crown to the base chakra, it serves as a reminder of others using TRT®.

"Using The Radiance Technique® in the hospice environment and to support my personal growth has encouraged a willingness to look at my own patterns of behaviour — not always a comfortable experience! I have found Front Position #1 particularly helpful when I am feeling angry or judgemental and Front Positions #2 and #3 when I am feeling unsure or fearful."

Areas of the body are reflected in the feet, hands and ears providing a map of the physical body. Reflexology promotes relaxation, balance, circulation and normalizes body functions. In conjunction with TRT®, it contributes to enhancing quality of life and a deeper connection in reflexology.

Michelle Lonsdale, a student of The Fifth Degree, also combines The Radiance Technique® with reflexology:

"I studied The First Degree Official Program of The Radiance Technique®, Authentic Reiki® in 1991 and over the years deepened my experience by taking further degrees," says Michelle. "I start and finish every day with hands-on and Attunements and continue them throughout the day. I feel that the Radiant energy permeates all my activities and keeps me strong on all levels.

"Nine years ago, I started giving sessions to adults who have learning disabilities and who live in communal households. Those people have no or little language, but communicate in their own way. The sessions consist of a combination of reflexology, metamorphic technique, and a short TRT® session at the end. I may direct symbols while doing the feet but more especially while I do TRT® and, of course, the Radiant energy flows through my hands while doing the feet because it flows all the time!

"I have noticed from the beginning that whether I do symbols or not, my presence creates a special atmosphere: in one house the two or three residents will congregate in the living room where I work and sit there happily while waiting for their turn, thus allowing their carers to get on with some work in the house. Two people actually make satisfied purring sounds when I start doing their heads. Some take their shoes off in anticipation and one autistic man will not have any other treatment. I feel that The Radiance Technique® creates a special energy even reaching out to the carers who, in some cases have to be present.

"This work is such a rewarding experience greatly magnified by TRT®, which enables me to connect at a very deep level with people who have limited communication skills and few opportunities for Radiant Touch®. My work did not have that magical element before The Radiance Technique®. I am so grateful to be able to give in this way and to receive so much in return."

Aromatherapy

Aromatherapy has been around for centuries assisting in wellness and in dying. The healing powers of aromas help calm the mind and relax the body. Wing Wei, in the 8th Century AD wrote, "Look in the perfumes of flowers and of nature for peace of mind and joy of life." The subtle nature of aromas helps in creating a healing environment.

Aromatherapy for the purposes of this book is using essential oils to assist in therapeutic benefits for patients and caregivers during their sessions of The Radiance Technique®. As a Certified Aromatherapist, I offer the following sugges- tions, which can be readily used by anyone and are mainly in the form of inhalation through diffuser or on a Kleenex. The number one rule to remember is that if a person does not like the scent, whatever it is, then don't use it. You want to avoid heavy perfume scents and most scented candles, plug-ins and incense, because those aromas are synthetic, adulterated and artificial. Most people have a respiratory or allergic reaction to them. Even standard hospital and home cleaning products/ fluids can be disturbing, along with most body products, hand soaps and perfumes.

The best way to purchase oils and candles is from a pro- fessional Aromatherapist or reputable distributor. It will cost more, but the quality is worth it. A trained nose knows.

One person I highly recommend is David Crow, L.Ac.. David has studied natural healing systems for more than twenty years. He is a licensed acupuncturist and herbalist who travels the world in search of certified organic and sus- tainably harvested essential oils, attars, hydrosols, natural perfumes and therapeutic formulations. David is the owner of Floracopeia® Aromatic Treasures and writes about one of the oldest forms of medicines in the world in his book, *In Search of the Medicine Buddha*, "Wafting through the olfactory chan- nels into the recesses of our ancestral brains, the mysteriously subtle and rightly complex smells of essential oils secreted by plants awaken memories, trigger positive alterations in mood, and stimulate immunity. Fragrance is the bridge connecting the colourfully scented plant realms, the human heart and soul, and the spheres of the gods."[1]

When I was receiving chemotherapy treatments, I remember how keen my sense of smell was. Chemo altered everything, even my taste buds. Before the medication was given to me, I could already taste it in my mouth. I also remember going into the bathroom in the Cancer Centre clinic and smelling the cleaning products that were used. It added to my stomach queasiness and nausea. Even when I completed my chemotherapy treatments and went to the clinic for my bi-monthly check-ups, the aroma in the bathroom immediately transported me back to my chemo days and gave me the same sick feelings even though I was not receiving chemotherapy. I learned another profound body-mind connection and how this aroma directly linked me to my past. Power of smell? Remembering? All correct. We have incredible brains with incredible powers. A friend suggested I put a dab of Vick's® VapoRub® under my nose so I would not smell the medication, and it worked.

Now when my clients experience feelings of nausea, I recommend the use of peppermint oil in a diffuser, or a few drops on a Kleenex for inhalation in combination with holding my hands on Head Positions #2 and #3 and Front Position #1 to help with discomfort.

I remember one patient from the Philippines. She would often share her love for flowers and how she missed the wonderful scent of ylang-ylang, the flower of the cananga tree. For her next Radiant Touch® visit, I surprised her, put a drop of the essential oil of ylang-ylang on a Kleenex, and asked her to inhale. A whole wave of memories came back to her of her childhood and during her session, she had many wonderful visualizations, including being back at home healthy and free of cancer.

I have used the scent of spearmint and rose in diffusers to bring joy to the heart and mind and an uplifting feeling. These oils can also be purchased in the form of spritzers and floral waters in a bottle, which you can spritz into a room, away from the client to change the aroma. Aromas are vibrations of scent as well and can assist in changing the mood of someone. Rose oil in particular has been supportive to caregivers experiencing loss and grief. The aroma of orange can also be uplifting. And with respect to the essential oil of lavender, of which there are over 200 different kinds, I tend to use *Lavandula angustafolia* for its relaxing and sedative properties. These familiar smells, along with reassuring touch of The Radiance Technique®, assist people in a better quality of life and enhanced well-being.

Aroma is not only beneficial for the client, but anyone coming into the room will benefit. I often find nurses smelling the aroma in the hallways and commenting how pleasant the room smells. Dr. Jane Buckle, Ph.D., R.N., writes in *Clinical Aromatherapy in Nursing* that, "Pleasant smells are of particular importance. The smell of death is something most nurses can recognize. Certainly if there are any fungating lesions, the smell in a patient's room can be quite unpleasant, and patients remain aware of both smell and touch almost until the end."[2]

There are also aromas that have been used over centuries to facilitate the dying process. One such oil is frankincense and another is the oil of oud. Oud is used by Tibetan and Ayurvedic doctors. David Crow, L.Ac., shares about the healing properties of this oil, "The effects of this rare and exquisite perfume on consciousness are so potent that it is used to open the doors between this world and the next, allowing the dying to pass peacefully into the afterlife."[3]

For native peoples, the four sacred medicines of sweet grass, sage, cedar and tobacco are used in ceremony for purification, cleansing and healing. These plants can be used singularly or a combination for smudging. Sweet grass is often used to smudge a dead person. I have also met shamans from South America that have used rose water to change the frequency of vibration. When appropriate, I have used these sacred medicines as well before or during a session of Radiant Touch®.

Scents like vanilla have been proven to have a calming affect, and this scent is used in some hospitals and clinics around Canada, the United States, and England. A simple candle placed in a safe area is subtle and can help with odours in the room. Just remember never to leave it unattended.

Healing Sounds

I have always been fascinated with the healing capacities of different dimensions of sound and its affect on my own healing. Everything around us in the universe and within us is in a state of vibration. Some of the most healing sounds are found in our natural world. There is even a new field known as *psychoacoustics* — the study of sound on humans. Sound frequency has a direct affect on how we feel and recover and researchers have concluded that the noise levels found on hospital wards can exceed the volume of a pneumatic drill. Don Campbell, the world's foremost educator on the connection between music and healing writes in his book, *The Mozart Effect*®, "Hospitals, one of the noisiest of environments, are also rediscovering the restorative value of quiet. Intensive care units, which are filled with the beeping of monitor alarms, the humming of motorized beds, and the pumping of ventilators, rank alongside airplane passenger cabins and factory floors as primary hazards to health and hearing. Preliminary research at the Medical College of Wisconsin in Milwaukee indicates that special noise-reduction earphones may speed up patient's healing."[4]

During my high school days, I remember hearing about the study of plants and music. The plants receiving rock music did not grow and often withered. When you are a teenager, such information does not have much effect while you are sharing time with your friends at a concert. I did remember observing how my friends' personalities changed while listening to hard rock, becoming more obnoxious, more daring and more rebellious. My personal study of sound and experience of sound over the years has changed my perspective as well as my taste for music. I became aware of my choices based on how I was feeling or what I needed in the moment. The following study conducted at The Ohio State University of the *Effect of Different Sounds on Growth of Human Cancer Cell Lines in Vitro* reveals, "Cells vibrate dynamically and may transmit information via harmonic waves motions. This study compared the effects of 'primordial sounds' (Sama Veda, from the Maharishi Ayur-Veda system of natural health care,) or hard rock music (AC/DC, 'Back in Black',) and no sound on the growth of cells in culture.... Primordial sound significantly decreased the average growth across cell lines (p=0.005)."[5]

I have included a selection of music in the Appendices that I have used with others and with myself during a TRT® session. We live in a technological, machine-aided age with the capability to bring every sound imaginable into our environment. In combination with hands-on or directing, the senses are invited to a deeper experience. Just remember that whatever you use, be open and flexible. What is music to your ears might not be to someone else's. It is always best to ask someone their preference and to keep in mind cultural sensitivity at all times.

However, if you have the opportunity, live natural sounds of water and birds are very healing. Live instrumental music which includes the harp, guitar, and violin, flute are also pleasing to the senses. Singing and vocal toning are also nurturing. That is why people go to concerts, attend live orchestra performances, sing at campfires or gravitate to areas of water and nature to experience vibrationally what machine-produced music cannot duplicate. Healing sounds cleanse, purify and bathe the spirit. The sounds of bells, rattles, native drums and Tibetan, crystal or wooden sounding bowls are very effective in having a direct vibrational effect on the physiology, mind and emotions and invite opportunities for communication.

For example, singing bowls are made of seven metals

and stimulate the body, including the brain, to rediscover its own harmonic frequency. The sounds are like an inner massage. Within these ancient sounds, the original harmonic frequency of life is recreated. I remember receiving a referral for a seven-year-old boy with a brain tumour who had trouble in his motor and communication skills after his operation. On my first visit for Radiant Touch®, I brought along two singing bowls, a small one four inches in diameter and a larger seven-inch bowl. With children, you need to be creative and interesting, and I used them to explain to Cody about vibration and what will happen in our session in a simple, interactive way. We practiced different exercises using this ancient sound therapy, and it was so amazing to witness his sensitivity of the sound. He would explain where the vibration travelled to different parts of his body, how it made him feel, and he just loved the wonderful sound it made. I was also teaching Cody how to do TRT® on himself, so this was a great introduction about vibration and what his hands could do. Over the next three months, he and I shared sessions together: I did his Head Positions, and he did his Front Positions. In between, with the singing bowl on his stomach, Cody would tap the bowl whenever he felt like it. He also described how he could feel movement throughout his body during his Radiant Touch® sessions. It was an incredible experience for me too. The Radiance Technique® itself is vibrational science, supporting in silence.

Kate Goulden, Complementary Therapist in a Hospice in Devon, England, illustrates the supportive qualities of combining TRT® with a wooden sounding bowl.

"As a complementary therapist working in a hospice environment I was privileged to be able to offer TRT® to one particular patient. This young man, a musician, was experiencing his dying process. Consciousness was variable, but he was able to indicate that he was comfortable with the idea of TRT® as a form of relaxation. His family members were supportive — I sensed that they were all on their own particular journey. The young man himself was a little like a shining beacon in the midst of his loving family. A chance presented itself to work with the music therapist using a sounding bowl, so that a combined TRT®/music session was offered. For me, the experience that followed highlighted the desirability of being able to offer, in the moment, care that had a truly holistic element. The room became for a while a still, quiet sanctuary. Simple hand movements in time to the music were a clear indication of the effect on the patient. Although we can never know, with certainty, the effect on the dying process of this kind of care, I was aware that all three of us present at that time experienced a sense of true connectedness."

The Power of Music

Music is a part of all of our lives and can play an important role during the journey. Vibrational tones are perceived by our outer senses and can alter moods, enhance feelings of self-worth and calm our body. It can invoke suppressed emotions, touch us deeply, and give permission to feel when we have no words. Sounds can also have a relieving effect on pain. Music and specific sound vibrations have been used in many cultures to activate healing, harmonize the mind-body, and connect to spirit.

Over the years, I heard and learned of other tones, especially Indian, Oriental and Tibetan, Laplander and native people's chants. These ancient sounds do not follow the seven-note scale I had learned on the piano in my youth. Many different forms of music employ direct body rhythm entrainment techniques. Ancient Indian classical music that I have used comes from the Gandharva Veda Music. There is a whole science about these particular musical melodies or *ragas* and how they relate directly to the frequency of different times of the day, our 24-hour body rhythms and the seasons. This music is in rhythm with nature and the natural laws of nature and has a harmonizing influence and balance of energy to bring peace, happiness and health in the whole body. I documented earlier the effects these sounds had on cancer cells. Maharishi Ayurveda Products International has a complete line of this type of music listed in the Appendices.

Debbie Danbrook's music induces relaxation and meditative benefits when brainwaves of the listener match the rhythms and sounds of the Shakuhachi bamboo flute. Debbie is a performer and composer who is a Master of the Japanese Shakuhachi, an ancient instrument originally played as a type of Zen. She is one of the first women in the world to master this difficult flute, traditionally only played by men. Debbie believes that music is an important part of the healing process, and she creates recordings that "heal the mind and soothe the soul." Her recent release, *Sacred Sounds of the Soul*, was created for her dying father. The music from this album is featured in the companion DVD of this book for its powerful sounds that generate inner reflection and peace to support the journey of the soul.

More modern versions of body rhythm entrainment techniques to synchronize the breath, heart and brain waves include the works of Dr. Lee Bartel in partnership with Somerset Entertainment, a leading producer and distributor of specialty music. Dr. Bartel is an Associate Professor and an Associate of the Centre for Health Promotion at the University of Toronto. He has taken his specialty of cognitive and emotional responses to music and created a whole series entitled, *Music for your Health*.

I was fascinated to read Paul Pearsall's groundbreaking book entitled, *The Heart's Code*, which explores many new findings about cellular memories and their role in the mind-body-spirit connection. He writes, "The energy of the heart, right down to our DNA is musical and rhythmic in nature."

He shares the findings of Geneticist Susumu Ohno of the Beckman Research Institute in Duarte, California who, "transcribed one of Chopin's musical passages to a chemical notation, the resulting formula resembled that of the DNA of a human cancer gene. It appears that even cancer cells have a memory for their own tune, one that is playing out of tune, too loud or too separately from the cellular orchestra. Ultimately, cancer may turn out to be a severe form of cellular disharmony caused by a section of the cellular symphony that has forgotten how to play with the rest of the group. Energy cardiology suggests that the heart is the conductor that keeps all the cells playing the same score."[6]

The health care field has come to know what cultures and traditions have for centuries — the power of music. Music therapy in palliative care has become a popular supportive care field of interest. For example, the Autumn 2001 *Journal of Palliative Care* devoted its entire issue to music. Music takes one where words can no longer be uttered. It can allow family members to remain actively involved through music and through song.

Using TRT® with music enhances the experience for all. It is important to observe that in the dying stages of one's life hearing is the last sense to go. Additionally, on-going practice of TRT® assists one in moving beyond ordinary perception, beyond ordinary hearing into deeper perceptions. Experiencing levels or planes of energy beyond our regular five senses is possible before the dying stages. I have, in my own study of TRT®, experienced moments of this clairaudience connecting me to my unlimited potential of deeper perception of myself and the world around me.

> *Music* — ...*In higher consciousness, transcendental vibrations can be heard by the Inner Ear as you awaken to and become a master of discerning Light vibrations of the Whole not audible with the outer ears. These sounds — these tonal*

vibrations of universal Light — are the radiant healing/ wholing power of harmonious alignment of the parts to the Whole. Nearly 24 centuries ago, the Greek philosopher Plato, an Initiate of the Egyptian Mystery Schools of Light, referred to this cosmic, transcendental Radiant sound woven within the very fabric of the universe as 'The Music of the Spheres.' [7]

Chanting, Toning and Healing Words

One of the most powerful instruments for healing is our voice. The voice has been used for centuries for healing and spiritual connection. My first introduction to voice was like all of us, making sounds when I was a baby, exploring my voice and the many dimensions of it. Later in life, somehow voice and sound became more structured and not as spontaneous. Over the years, I have been drawn to explore sounds, in particular, my voice, and learned more about the benefits of toning and history of chanting from author and pioneer of sound healing, Jill Purce. Author of *The Mystic Spiral*, Jill teaches people to find their healing voice through ancient vocal techniques. She studied many traditions over the years including the Gyuto Tibetan Monastery and Tantric College learning forms of Mongolian and Tibetan chanting. Jill says, "If you can use sound to work on the morphogenetic field of the person, in other words the resonant potentiality of their own healthy state, then you can maintain that person in a state of health. In language to be healthy is to be sound — we talk about being sound in body and mind, to be of sound mind and to have ideas which ring true. I work at this level to try and tune the instrument which the human being is. To maintain a person in tune is to maintain them in a state of health." [8]

I use Jill's teachings of chanting and overtone chanting and incorporate them with The Radiance Technique®. It is an incredible expansion when both are used in combination.

Vocal toning is finding your healing voice through sound. There are a number of Authorized Instructors of The Radiance Technique® who teach specialized courses using TRT® for vocal expansion and healing. One of my teachers is Ingrid St Clare. Her interest and delight in the human voice led to her special focus teaching voice and speech at Drama Schools in California and London, England. She combines TRT® with all her work and told me that my voice is supported by many components: my posture, my tone, and my breath. She said that the most relaxing breath is through exhaling and suggests the following TRT® positions for supporting the breath: Front Positions #1, 2, 3 and Back Positions #1, 2, and 3. A whole book could be written on this subject; I am only briefly touching upon it in this book.

There are many health benefits of sounding vowels, the ones you learned in your early years of school. If teachers only knew the powerful potential of vowel sounds that went beyond speaking and reading the vowels, it would certainly bring a new dimension to learning and healing. Ingrid St Clare uses vocal toning by combining with TRT® in her *Voice and Movement* workshops. Try the following simple combination for vocal exploration:

RADIANT TONING EXERCISE

Begin with the vowel sounds of A, E, I, O, U sounding as AH, EH, E, O, U.

- Sit in a comfortable chair with your hands on Head Position #4.
- Close your eyes and simply observe your breath flowing in and out of your body.
- Next take in a gentle breath and on your exhalation, tone the vowel A as "AH" as if you are singing one

musical note. It does not matter what note, any one that would be easy and comfortable for you. It also does not matter how loud or long it is. Sustain the vowel to the end of your breath then take a break of one complete breath and try again.

- During this process you can move your hands to Front Position #1.
- The vowel sounds correspond to the third eye, throat, heart, naval and spine respectively.
- If you have studied advanced degrees of TRT®, incorporating the Cosmic Symbols with your toning will enhance the experience. You can also invite others to join in while you are doing hands-on as well.
- When beginning, do not overdue it, as you might get light headed.
- As you practice and feel at ease, begin to find your own voice that is unique to you.

Mantras

Sounds such as AUM and OM are ancient with their own interior vibratory properties.

Mantra — A sound based on systems of vibrations which access higher energies and support the student for higher consciousness and spiritual awakening. Although Eastern vibratory sciences are interrelated, each has its own component parts and processes. The Radiance Technique® within its interior processes is not comprised of a mantra system but rather of universal energy symbols. The Radiance Technique® can be used to enhance and expand a mantra facilitating the opening and awakening of consciousness.[9]

As shared above by Dr. Barbara Ray, mantras are beyond uttering words or vowels and are in a category all by themselves. They are sacred tones or sounds in ancient languages.

Some can affect certain illnesses or help clear your mind; others connect you to a lineage of teachers and their attainment. The latter type is explained by Gehlek Rimpoche, "Mantras are road maps in helping one transform. They have a different quality when one receives initiations... The word mantra is mind protection and affects the mind, influences and changes mind's way of thinking and functioning. In addition to that it has its own supernatural power which affects us, environment, affects air and where air travels... it has unlimited power and the power to enlighten."[10]

I have used in my own practice reciting mantras in conjunction with my TRT® meditations. Bringing the two together does in fact expand my personal capacities for inner sight, inner hearing and inner feeling.

Hypnotherapy and Visualization

Van Ault wrote the first book and produced the first video on how hypnosis and the loving touch of transcendental energy actually work together. His book, *Hypnotherapy and The Radiance Technique®: Partners in Transformation*, details the dynamic connection and expansion therapists and clients can experience with this combination. Van felt that TRT® enabled him to move beyond both the conscious and subconscious levels of the psyche that hypnosis alone cannot reach.

In a typical induction, Van incorporates hands-on Head Positions #2 and #3, as he explains,

Feel your head relaxing: the top of your head, the back of your neck, your face — and allow this relaxation to move through the rest of your body, as you continue breathing deeply.... From there, the induction can go through relaxing the rest of the body or take some other course. Some clients go so deeply and so rapidly into trance that it's really a waste of time to lengthen the induction. So I go directly on to other work, but no matter how the hypnotic journey is timed, I insist on a minimum of five minutes of hands-on with each position, as is the standard practice with TRT.[11]

There are universal techniques in prayer, imagery and self-healing visualizations to improve quality of life, and many teachings found in religions have strong meditative traditions. They can improve white-blood cell response, affect pulse rate, normalize blood pressure, and balance stress hormone levels. In his revealing book, *Healing Words*, Larry Dossey, M.D., explores the efficacy of prayer and research done over the years.

When I was first diagnosed, Kate Kent, Dip.Ac., C.H., gave me the book, *Love, Medicine and Miracles*. In it, I learned a lot about creating a healing partnership with myself and with others, and began practicing visualization techniques. I actually wrote to Dr. Bernie Siegel back in 1989, thanking him for the inspiration revealed in his book, and I was surprised to receive a hand-written letter back from him. I still have the letter he wrote in purple ink, *Dear Christine, With acceptance comes peace of mind and the ability to heal oneself. Peace, Bernie.* Since that time, he has written more books and produced wonderful CD's and tapes for mental imagery and visualization.

Visualization is often directed toward a specific goal, like seeing oneself healthy where imagery is more about feeling. According to Bernie Siegel, M.D., "From years of experience in using the visualization technique we do know that the image must be chosen by the individual. It must be an image that the person can see in the mind's eye as clearly as something seen by the physical eye. It must be an image with which the patient feels completely comfortable."[12]

I encourage patients during their sessions of TRT® to feel free to incorporate affirmations, imagery or prayer. Used in combination, deeper states of awareness are possible. It can be supportive to create images that are positive, instead of focusing on doom and gloom. In the eighties, Pac-Man was a popular video game, and I had utilized the suggestions for the book, *Getting Well Again*, in visualizing and drawing these

Pac-Man figures eating up the cancer in my body and leaving the good cells.

Using the above techniques is useful and helpful, but sometimes limited. When one is unable to concentrate or visualize, these techniques are essentially unavailable. They are mind exercises that arise from memories and imagination. Having TRT® as a tool is unique because it is a method that bypasses the mind and can give rise to deeper levels of inner awareness that are different from the experience of visualization as Dr. Barbara Ray explains:

> *Visualize, Visualization* — *Refers to the formation of a mental image or vision of. The Radiance Technique® is not a mental technique or a technique using visualizing or visualization at <u>any level</u>. The Radiance Technique® accesses universal, transcendental, whole energy directly which promotes from <u>within</u> awareness of all the inner senses — inner sight, inner hearing, inner touch, inner smell, and inner taste. Ongoing and daily applications of The Radiance Technique® support your growth in higher consciousness and expand the development of the capacities for 'seeing' from within with the inner eye. This process is different from visualization where the image is being <u>recreated </u>through the use of the mental plane. ...*[13]

Many people have shared with me that in their TRT® sessions, they see images, colours, and create their own visualizations spontaneously, as some have described in this book. Many have also received confirmation or clarity about an issue or problem they have been dealing with. One particular patient was a woman in her late 60s who was diagnosed with lymphatic cancer and learned a year later that it had spread throughout her body. She explained:

"I experienced total relaxation, my muscles relaxed, and my breathing was easier. My mind relaxed. I had visions to enter, encouragement to stay in touch with my body, to listen and to feel."

Nina loved the ocean, and we would use this sound during our sessions. A particularly potent visualization came to her on my last visit with her. Nina described herself as floating peacefully in the ocean, observing the coral in the polluted water and that it was slowly dying. She said halfway through her TRT® session, the current changed, restoring the coral to "full living beauty." Full living beauty echoed over and over again as I learned of her transition two days later.

When engaging in visualization, I recommend hands-on just before and during it. I have supported patients combining visualization with their TRT® session, especially when people have a difficult time in relaxing their mind at the beginning of the session. If it is a tape you are listening to, spend about 20 minutes on the four Head Positions and then turn the tape on. Your body and mind will be more relaxed and the healing process will have already begun. The daily chatter of our mind and the negative thoughts and emotions can be very draining on all aspects of our being. TRT® can be used in conjunction with positive words and affirmations to go deeper into the negative imprints of ourselves and heal them from within, not just from the mental mind. Patients, caregivers and others can use the suggestions offered by Dr. Barbara Ray for expanding the healing potential of ourselves.

Affirmations — May be written down and said aloud and are especially enhanced when combined with this radiant, universal energy as a cosmic support for your true unfolding process. Always use words that convey the deeper energy principles you wish to manifest in your life. Transformative energies are amplified when the hands are used over the heart center in Front Position #1 while saying daily affirmations. It is very supportive to create your own affirmations that support your movement from the known of where you are to the unknown of the direction in which you wish to go. For example, 'I am becoming a loving person,' is an affir-

mation that can grow within you as you say it aloud and within yourself throughout the day. Placing your hands at the heart center supports the unconditional self to respond from the inner dimensions. 'I am growing and transforming' is an affirmation that can build a bridge for you to that unknown that occurs in the process of growth and consciousness expanding. It is also effective to create your own affirmations and expand them as you move into new ways of being.[14]

A wonderful meditation/visualization that I have used is known as *Loving Kindness Meditation*. This and other meditations found in Stephen Levine's book *Healing into Life and Death* can be used along with Radiant Touch®. There are many versions, and the one below is a popular version from Stephen Levine that has also been put to music in the CD entitled, *Songs of Healing*.

Use TRT® to deepen your capacities for compassion and unconditional love toward yourself and toward others. You may begin with your hands on your Heart Centre, Front Position #1, and say :

"May I dwell in the heart.
May I be free of suffering.
May I be healed.
May I be at peace."[15]

Then you can modify the words and replace "I" with someone else's name.

There is also an entry in *The Expanded Reference Manual of The Radiance Technique®, Authentic Reiki®*:

Blessings — ... *'Today, I will count my many blessings,' is a supportive way to affirm all of the parts of your wholeness that contribute to your well-being, your sense of wholeness and harmony. While using the hands-on application of The*

Radiance Technique, you can interrelate this affirmation and create others while your hands are in different positions such as Front Position #1, the Heart Center, to explore deeper ways of knowing your blessings on a daily basis. Expand your awareness by noting in your journal your observations as you apply this radiant energy.[16]

The following is a non-denominational prayer that can be used for personal expansion.

Prayer Treatment For Receptivity

There is one divine power, which is Love, Joy, and Abundance... awake and omnipresent in all life. I know that I am connected to this power. I acknowledge its presence in this universe, and I welcome its playful creativity in my world. Right here and right now, I align with this one power of love.

And through this power, I claim that I am receptive to the treasures of the universe. Like a flower unfolding in sunlight, I receive the life-giving rays of my spiritual source. I am willing to accept all the blessings, gifts, and energy that are intended for me today. I allow my heart to blossom with divine prosperity, divine creativity, and divine harmony in all its forms! I also claim that any negative, constricting beliefs about myself or the nature of the universe are overridden this instant by the law of love. I can receive now, and I can give now, from the spirit of universal joy.

I accept that my receptivity to love has expanded, and continues to stretch from this moment on. I embrace the generosity that I can also share with others. Nothing can stop the universe from generating its abundance in my life right this instant! With gratitude to that radiant, eternal source within me, I give thanks that this is done, and I let it be. And so it is!

~Van R. Ault, 1993[17]

There are unlimited possibilities to integrate transcendental energy with your daily activities at work, home, school or volunteer service. Radiant energy in your inner and outer environments helps you to be in touch with your inner source of life.

It is with deep honour to have the opportunity to share with you healing moments along life's journey. Experiences with The Radiance Technique® have given me a deeper inner knowing of myself within my own cycles of wellness and illness and have 'lightened up' my perception of death and dying. In the stillness of silence or in a gentle touch, I know that The Radiance Technique® supports my awakening journey with Real Light. I hope the personal stories have touched your heart and illuminated a deeper awareness within you.

May this book open you to the possibilities of what life is. Appreciate your timeless nature and the preciousness of your life Here Now.

~ *Christine*

[1] David Crow, *In Search of the Medicine Buddha: A Himalayan Journey*, (New York, NY: Tarcher/Putnam, 2000), p. 174.

[2] Jane Buckle, RN, *Clinical Aromatherapy in Nursing*, (London, England: Singular Publishing Group, 1997), p. 229.

[3] Crow, *In Search of the Medicine Buddha: A Himalayan Journey*, p. 175.

[4] Don Campbell, *The Mozart Effect®*, (New York, NY: Avon Books, 1997), p. 38.

[5] "Effect of Different Sounds on Growth of Human Cancer Cell Lines In Vitro," Alternative Therapies in Clinical Practice, Vol. 3, No. 4, pp. 25-32, 1996.

[6] Paul Pearsall, M.D., The Heart's Code, (New York, NY: Broadway Books 1999), p. 102.

[7] Ray, *The Expanded Reference Manual of The Radiance Technique®, Authentic Reiki®*, (St. Petersburg, FL: Radiance Associates, 1987), p. 72.

[8] Jill Purce, Sound in Mind and Body, *Resurgence Magazine* No. 115 March/April 1986.

[9] Ray, *The Expanded Reference Manual of The Radiance Technique®, Authentic Reiki®*, p. 69.

[10] Gehlek Rimpoche, Ann Arbor Jewel Heart *Joyful Summer Retreat 2003*, Albion, Michigan.

[11] Ault, Van, *Hypnotherapy and The Radiance Technique®: Partners in Transformation*, (San Francisco, CA: Resources for Renewal, 1992), p. 27-29.

[12] Bernie Siegel, M.D., *Love, Medicine and Miracles*, (New York, NY: Harper & Row Publishers, 1986), p. 155.

[13] Ray, *The Expanded Reference Manual of The Radiance Technique®, Authentic Reiki®*, p. 114.

[14] *Ibid.*, p. 8.

[15] Stephen Levine, *Healing into Life and Death*, (New York, NY: Anchor Books, 1987), p. 23.

[16] Ray, *The Expanded Reference Manual of The Radiance Technique®, Authentic Reiki®*, p. 16.

[17] From the writings of Van R. Ault, 1993. Reprinted with permission of Cathie Ault-Kash Family.

Acknowledgments

This book and companion DVD was a worldwide community effort made possible by the loving support of many contributors who were willing to devote time and energy to share their experiences.

Gratitude for the support and encouragement from:

- Van R. Ault — my inspiration, my friend.
  Deep gratitude to you for encouraging me to become a teacher of TRT® and to write my experiences.
- The entire Hospice Radiant Touch® Volunteer Team.
- Contributing authors of this book.
- Patients and caregivers who graciously allowed me to share moments of their life's journey.
- The various readers who helped with editing including Marvelle Lightfields, Fred W. Wright Jr., Katherine Lenel, Shoshana Shay, Ann Healy, Ingrid St Clare, Maya Melrose, Marty Gervais, Joe Kornowski, Marie Jeanette, Sarah St. Pierre and Debbie Johnson.
- The layout, typesetting and design of the book and DVD cover under the creative eye of Meredith Karns, of *Morgan Meredith Inc.*
- The final DVD production team under the creative and professional direction of Pat Jeflyn and Kim Kristy of *Canadian Arts Productions.*
- Angelo Verrelli of *Visual Expression Photography & Video* and Andrea Slavik of *House of Toast* for additional footage and support.

Ongoing support and encouragement from: Tina Gross, Traugott Gross, Ray Imai, Ilse Hafenstein, Dr. Paul Dugliss, Mary Rose Bearfoot-Jones, Gerry Nagle, Dr. Delores Sicari, Dr. Abu-Zahra, Dr. Tom Barnard, Mary-Jo Rusu, Ayurveda colleagues, Hospice staff and board of directors and my many friends and family for their caring gestures, inspiration and love.

Generous Donations from:

- Courtney Milne and Sherrill Miller of Courtney Milne Productions Inc. — Cover Photograph
- Morgan Meredith Inc. — Design and Typesetting

Financial and Promotional Support provided by the following families and supporters:

- The Bachand Family
- The Dennis Family
- The Gorski Family
- The Gross Family
- The Hidalgo Family
- The Imperoli Family
- The Karns Family
- The Koch-Donga Family
- Family and Friends of Ann McCloud
- The Pollock Family
- The Rogin Family
- The Sikkema Family
- The Vitti Family
- Dr. Thomas J. Barnard and Sarah Shapiro
- In Honour of the Ones We Love Inc.
- Maximizing People Potential
- Dr. Zoia Sherman
- The Hospice of Windsor and Essex County Inc.
- The Radiance Technique International Association, Inc.
- The United Way of Windsor Essex County
- Valiant Machine & Tool Inc.
- Windsor Regional Hospital

Appendices

ENERGY MODEL
Vibrational Planes of Energy   Spectrum of Consciousness
Transforming – Wholing Process

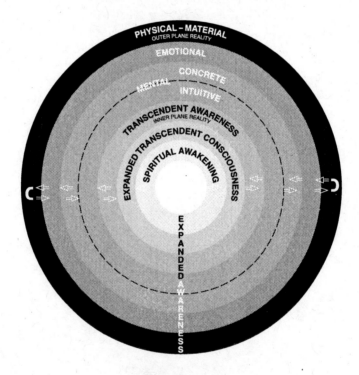

INNER TO OUTER
DENSITY TO ENLIGHTENMENT

For Information on books and resources about
The Radiance Technique®, Authentic Reiki®and
about The Radiant TRT Heart First Ashram®
Healing/Wholing Network:

The Radiance Technique
International Association, Inc.
(TRTIA)

P.O. Box 40570
St. Petersburg, Florida 33743 USA

Telephone/Fax: 727-347-2106
Email: TRTIA@aol.com
Web Site: www.trtia.org

International TRT ® Associations

La Associazione Radiance Technique® Italiana Real Reiki-Milano
Via G. Pascoli, 3
20129 Milano
ITALY

Die Radiance Technik Gesellschaft e.V. (DRTG)
Hobrechtstr. 67/Aufgang 2
12047 Berlin
GERMANY
drtg-ev@t-online.de

The Radiance Technique Association for Great Britain
(TRTAGB)
7 Park House, Park Drive
Market Harborough,
Leicestershire LE16 7BS
ENGLAND
TRTAGB@aol.com

Verein der Radiance Technik® Österreich
Millergasse 24A/3
1060 Wien
AUSTRIA

Website with Partial List of Authorized Instructors
www.AuthenticReiki.org

Book Contributors who are TRT®Authorized Instructors:

Austria
Miki Ivancsics
  office@energietraining.at
  www.energietraining.at

Canada
Pat Bachand
  pat.bachand@sympatico.ca
Melanie Johnson
  RadiantOneMJ@yahoo.ca

Germany
Brigitte Strobel, Berlin
  radiant.sunshine@freenet.de
Leslie Christopher
  info@trtnursing.com
Ulrike Wolf, Berlin
  Ulrike.Wolf@t-online.de

Great Britain
Maya Melrose
  maya@livingful.co.uk
Ingrid St Clare
  istclare@phonecoop.coop

USA

Dawn Champion, Florida & USA
trtchampion@msn.com

Leslie Christopher, Washington & USA
info@trtnursing.com

Joyce Kenyon, California & USA
RadiantJK@radiant-healinghands.com
www.radiant-healinghands.com

Marvelle Lightfields
lfields77@aol.com

Linda Richard, Arizona
LRichard37@acn.net

Marcia Ward, Oklahoma
starmar42@earthlink.net

Fred W. Wright Jr.
TravelWord@aol.com

For information about Authorized Instructors, seminars, and The Advanced Degrees of The Radiance Technique®:
Radiance Seminars, Inc.
P.O. Box 7088
Seminole, Florida 33775 U.S.A.
RSIRadiantPeace@gmail.com

To contact the author, Christine Maria Gross, email:
portalwisdom7@gmail.com

©

For Information on
The Hospice ofWindsor and
Essex County Inc.

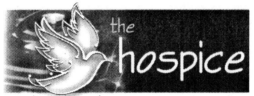

The Hospice of Windsor and Essex County Inc.
L'Hospice de Windsor-Essex Inc.

6038 Empress Street
Windsor, Ontario
N8T 1B5
Canada

Telephone: 519-974-7100
Web Site: www.thehospice.ca

Cover photo donated by world-renowned photographer

COURTNEY MILNE

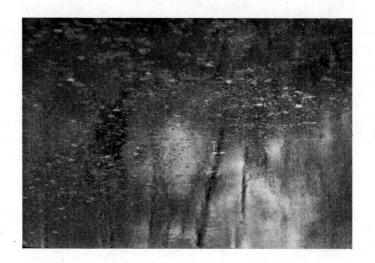

"The photographs I feel inspired to create,

from a place of unconditional love,

bring healing to both our inner

and outer landscapes"

Box 121
Grandora, Saskatchewan
S0K 1V0
Canada

306.668.1399
www.courtneymilne.com

On-Line Resources

The Radiance Technique®

www.trtia.org — The Radiance Technique International Association, Inc.

www.AuthenticReiki.org — Partial List of Authorized Instructors

Wellness

www.CaliforniaIntegrativeMedicine.com — Centre for Wellness and Integrative Medicine

www.commonweal.org — Commonweal Cancer Help Program and Retreats

www.ecap-online.org — Dr. Bernie Siegel EcaP (Exceptional Cancer Patients)

www.healingjourney.ca — Dr. Alastair Cunningham (The Healing Journey Program)

www.healingvoice.com — Jill Purce, International Healing Sound Movement Pioneer

www.pmri.org — The Preventive Medicine Research Institute

www.mbmi.org — Bensen-Henry Institute for Mind Body Medicine

www.willow.org — Willow Breast Cancer Support

www.cbcn.ca — Canadian Breast Cancer Network

www.cancer.ca — Canadian Cancer Society

www.cancerproject.org — The Cancer Project

www.realtimecancer.org — Cancer Support for Young Adults

www.cwhn.ca — Canadian Women's Health Network

www.plwc.org — People Living With Cancer — American Society of Clinical Oncology

Ayurveda Resources

www.drdugliss.com — Dr. Paul Dugliss
www.newworldayurveda.com
www.mapi.com — Maharishi Ayurveda

Tibetan Resources

www.tibetan-medicine.org — Tibetan Medical & Astro.
Institute of H. H. the Dalai Lama
www.jewelheart.org — Jewel Heart — Gelek Rimpoche
www.fpmt.org — The Foundation for the Preservation of the
Mahayana Tradition

Aromatherapy

www.floracopeia.com — David Crow L.Ac./Floracopeia®
www.rjbuckle.com — Dr. Jane Buckle
www.cfacanada.com — Can. Federation of Aromatherapists
www.naha.org — National Assoc. of Holistic Aromatherapy

Reflexology

www.reflexologycanada.ca — RAC
www.rrco-reflexology.com — RRCO

Hospice

www.centerforloss.com — Dr. Alan Wolfelt
www.davidkessler.org — David Kessler
www.growthhouse.org — Growth House Inc.
www.chpca.net — The Canadian Hospice Palliative Care Assoc.
www.hospicecare.com — International Assoc. for Hospice
and Palliative Care
www.hospicenet.org — For Patients and Families Facing
Life-Threatening Illness
www.hospice.on.ca — Ontario Hospice Association
www.spcare.org — Spiritual Care Program International
www.upaya.org — Upaya Institute and Zen Center
www.virtualhospice.ca — Canadian Virtual Hospice

Suggested Reading

Ault, Van R. *Hypnotherapy and The Radiance Technique®*. San Francisco, CA: Resources For Renewal, 1992.

Ault, Van R. *The Radiance Technique® and AIDS*. San Francisco, CA: Resources for Renewal, 1995.

Ballentine, Rudolph, M.D. *Radical Healing*. New York, NY: Harmony Books, 1999.

Bensen, Herbert, M.D. *Timeless Healing*. New York, NY: Scribner, 1996.

Bernay, Tony, Ph.D., and Porrath, Saar, M.D. *When It's Cancer: The 10 Essential Steps to Follow After Your Diagnosis*. USA: Rodale Inc., 2006.

Byock, Ira, M.D. *The Four Things That Matter Most: A Book About Living*. New York, NY: Free Press, Simon & Schuster, Inc., 2004.

Buckle, Jane, RN. *Clinical Aromatherapy in Nursing*, 1st Edition. London, England: Singular Publishing Group, 1997.

Callanan, Maggie, and Kelley, Patricia. *Final Gifts*. New York, NY: Schribner, 2000.

Carrington, Yesnie. *The Radiance Technique®, Authentic Reiki®: Empowerment and Wellbeing Strategies with Surgery and Related Experiences*. Golden, CO: Carrington, 2006.

Chopra, Deepak, M.D. *Ageless Body, Timeless Mind: The Quantum Alternative to Growing Old*, New York, NY: Harmony Books, 1993.

Coberly, Margaret, Ph.D., RN. *Sacred Passage: How to Provide Fearless, Compassionate Care for the Dying*. Boston, Mass: Shambhala Publications Inc., 2002.

Cunningham, Alastair J., O.C., Ph.D. *The Healing Journey: Overcoming the Crisis of Cancer*. Toronto, ON: Key Porter Books Ltd., 1992, 2000.

His Holiness the Dalai Lama. *Advice on Dying and Living a Better Life*. New York, NY: Atria Books, 2002.

Dass, Ram, and Bush, Mirabai. *Compassion in Action. Setting Out on the Path of Service*. New York, NY: Bell Tower, 1992.

Dossey, Larry, M.D. *Healing Beyond the Body*. Boston, Massachusetts: Shambhala Publications, 2001.

Dowling Singh, Kathleen. *The Grace in Dying*. New York, NY: HarperCollins, 1998.

Dugliss, Paul, M.D. *Ayurveda — The Power to Heal*, Michigan: MDC Publications, 2008.

Halifax, Joan, Ph.D. *Being with Dying: Cultivating Compassion and Fearlessness in the Presence of Death*. Boston, MA: Shambhala Publications Inc., 2008

Halpern, Steven. *Sound Health*. New York: Harper & Row, 1985.

Hanh, Thich Nhat. *No death, No fear. Comforting Widsom for Life*. New York, NY: Riverhead Books, 2002.

Keltie, Anne. *The Radiance Technique® And Death And Dying, A Journey in Awakening*. Kingsbury, London, Great Britain: Anne Keltie, 1995.

Kessler, David. *The Needs of the Dying: A Guide For Bringing Hope, Comfort, and Love to Life's Final Chapter*. New York, NY: HarperCollins, 2001.

Kubler-Ross, Elisabeth, and Kessler, David. *On Grief and Grieving: Finding The Meaning of Grief Through the Five Stages of Loss*. New York, NY: Scribner, 2005.

Kubler-Ross, Elisabeth, and Kesler, David. *Life Lessons*. New York, NY: Scribner, 2000.

Kuhl, David, M.D. *What Dying People Want: Practical Wisdom for the End of Life*. Canada: Doubleday, 2002.

Lenel, Katherine. *The Radiance Technique® And Cancer*. St. Petersburg, FL.: TRTAI, 1994.

Levine, Stephen. *A Year to Live*. New York, NY: Bell Tower, 1997.

Lightfields, Marvelle. *The Radiance Technique® and The Animal Kingdom*. St. Petersburg, FL.: Radiance Associates, 1992.

Longaker, Christine. *Facing Death and Finding Hope*. New York, NY: Main Street Books Doubleday, 1997.

Matthews-Simonton, Stephanie and Simonton, M.D., O. Carl. *Getting Well Again*. New York, NY: Bantam Books, 1984.

Montagu, Ashley. Touching. *The Human Significance of the Skin*. New York, NY: Harper & Row, 1971.

Ontario Multifaith Council on Spiritual and Religious Care. *Multifaith Information Manual*. Toronto, Ontario: Ontario Multifaith Council, 2002.

Pearce, Joseph Chilton. *The Biology of Transcendence. A Blueprint of the Human Spirit*. Rochester, Vermont: Inner Traditions International, 2002.

Pearsall, Paul, Ph.D. *The Heart's Code*. New York, NY: Random House, 1998.

Quinn, Rick. Terminal Diagnosis. *Help for the newly diagnosed cancer patient and those who love them*. Windsor, Ontario: Benchmark Publishing and Design Inc., 2002.

Ray, Barbara, Ph.D. *The 'Reiki' Factor in The Radiance Technique®*. St. Petersburg, FL.: Radiance Associates, 1992.

Ray, Barbara, Ph.D. *The Expanded Reference Manual of The Radiance Technique® A-Z*. St. Petersburg, FL.: Radiance Associates, 1987.

Ray, Barbara, Ph.D. *The Official Handbook of The Radiance Technique®, Authentic Reiki®, Updated Expanded Edition*. St. Petersburg, FL.: The Radiance Technique International Association, Inc. and Radiance Seminars, Inc., 2007.

Ray, Barbara, Ph.D. *The Radiance Technique® and Managing*

Stress. St. Petersburg, FL.: Radiance Associates, 1994.

Ray, Barbara, Ph.D. with Shoshana Shay, comp. *'This Moment in Time,' The Awakening Journey® Day by Day, Selecttions from the Teachings of Dr. Barbara Ray.* St. Petersburg, FL.: Radiance Associates, 2002.

Remen, Rachel Naomi, M.D. *Kitchen Table Wisdom.* New York, NY: Riverhead Books, 1996.

Rimpoche, Nawang Gehlek. *Good Life, Good Death: Tibetan Wisdom on Reincarnation.* New York, NY: Riverhead Books, 2001.

Rinpoche, Sogyal. *The Tibetan Book of Living and Dying.* San Francisco, CA: HarperCollins, 1994.

Siegel, Bernie S., M.D. Peace, *Love & Healing.* New York, NY: Harper Perennial, 1989.

Stone, Ganga. *Start the Conversation,* New York, NY: Warner Books Inc., 1996.

Wright, Jr., Fred. *The Radiance Technique® On The Job.* St. Petersburg, FL.: Radiance Associates, 1992.

Wolf, Ulrike. *Die Radiance Technik®: Das authentische Reiki®,* München, Germany: Goldman Verlag.,1999.

Yarema, Thomas R., M.D., and Rhonda, Daniel, and Brannigan, Johnny. *Eat Taste Heal: An Ayurvedic Cookbook for Modern Living.* Kapaa, Hawaii: Five Elements Press, 2006.

Yogananda, Paramahansa. *Scientific Healing Affirmations,* Los Angeles, CA: Self- Realization Fellowship, 1990.

Suggested Music
On-Line Resources

www.healingmusic.com — Music of Debbie Danbrook
- Debbie's music is featured in companion DVD of this book
- *Sacred Sounds for the Soul*
- *Sacred Sounds for Sleep*
- *Miracles*

www.somersetent.com — Somerset Entertainment
- Offers a line of music that takes people on sound journeys combining music and nature sounds

Any CD's from the "*Music for Your Health Collection*"
- *Natural Sleep Inducement*
- *Natural Relaxation*
- *Stream of Dreams*
- *Soothing Surf*
- *Rhythms of the Sea*
- *Pachelbel Forever by the Sea*
- *Cradle Classics*

www.audioshop.living-dying.com — Graceful Passages

www.emeraldharp.com — Christina Tourin's website

www.innerpeacemusic.com — Steven Halpern

www.mapi.com — Gandharva Veda Music

www.mozarteffect.com — Don Campbell

www.sound-remedies.com — Sound Remedies

www.soundstrue.com — Sounds True Music

CDs

Chakra Suite, Music for Sound Healing, In the Key of Healing, Accelerating Self-Healing by Steven Halpern

Chakra Delight: Singing Bowls for Balancing the Energy Centres — Book and CD, Binkey Kok Publications, Hofstede DeWeide Hoek — Havelte/Holland, 2001.

Dreamland by Scott Fitzgerald and Richard Hooper, World Disc Productions

JourneySongs by Michael Stillwater

Melody for Celebration and Joyfulness by Shir Kumar Sharma, from mapi.com

Miracles by Robert Whitesides-Woo

Starlight by Christina Tourin

Overtone Chanting Meditations — by Jill Purce

Prescriptions for Stress Sound Medicine™ Series — Instrumental Music with Brain Wave Tones, Kokopelli Recording Company, 2002.

Shepherd Moons by Enya, Reprise Records, Warner Music, 1991.

Seven Metals — Singing Bowls of Tibet by Benjamin Iobst, 1999.

Songs of Healing, Alleluia, Kyrie by On Wings of Song and Robert Gass — Spring Hill Music, 1992.

Wind & Mountain, Reiki, Buddha Nature by Deuter

Guided Meditation CDs

Graceful Passages: A Companion for Living and Dying by Michael Stillwater and Gary Malkin, — is an audio CD containing music with spoken passages from a variety of spiritual leaders and leaders in end-of-life care.

Healing Waterfall I and II by Max Highstein with Jill Andre

Letting Go of Stress with Dr. Emmett E. Miller, M.D., www. drmiller.com

Prescriptions for Living — Meditations by Dr. Bernie S. Siegel, M.D.

The Healing Voice — Lecture and Meditation by Jill Purce

The Peace Garden of Color — CD for children of all ages, www.peacegardenofcolor.com

The Companion DVD
We Are Timeless: The Radiance Technique® in Hospice Care
features the music of

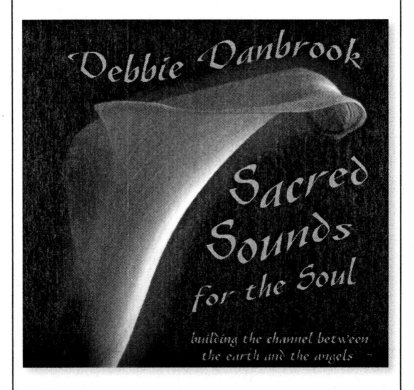

'Sacred Sounds for the Soul'
is one of the Healing Music recordings of
Debbie Danbrook. Debbie is a Shakuhachi Master,
the first woman to have mastered this
ancient Zen Japanese flute.

www.healingmusic.com

Permissions

The following authors and publishers have generously given permission to use extended quotations from copyrighted works:

From *The Expanded Reference Manual of The Radiance Technique®, Authentic Reiki®, Expanded Edition* by Barbara Ray, Ph.D. Copyright © 1987 by Dr. Barbara Ray. Used by permission from Dr. Barbara Ray.

From *The 'Reiki' Factor in The Radiance Technique® Expanded Edition* by Barbara Ray, Ph.D. Copyright © 1983,1985,1988,1992 by Dr. Barbara Ray. Used by permission from Dr. Barbara Ray.

From *'This Moment in Time,' The Awakening Journey® Day by Day* by Dr. Barbara Ray with Shoshana Shay, comp. Copyright © 2002 by Barbara Ray, Ph.D. Used by permission from Dr. Barbara Ray and Shoshana Shay.

From *The Radiance Technique® and AIDS* by Van R. Ault. Copyright © 1995 Van R. Ault. Used by permission from The Radiance Technique International Association, Inc.

From *Hypnotherapy and The Radiance Technique®: Partners in Transformation* by Van R. Ault. Copyright © 1992 Van R. Ault. Used by permission from The Radiance Technique International Association, Inc.

From the private writings of Van R. Ault, 1993. Reprinted with permission of Cathie Ault-Kash Family.